# WELLNESS ON A SHOESTRING

Seven Habits for a Healthy Life

# WELLNESS ON A SHOESTRING

## Seven Habits for a Healthy Life

**Michelle Robin, D.C.,**
**and**
**Roxanne Renée Grant**

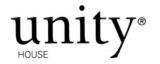

HOUSE

Unity Village, MO 64065-0001

*Wellness on a Shoestring*

First Edition 2010

Unity House books are available at special discounts for bulk purchases for study groups, book clubs, sales promotions, book signings or fundraising. To place an order, call the Unity Customer Care Department at 1-800-251-3571 or e-mail *sales@unityonline.org*.

Cover design: Jenny Hahn

Interior design: The Covington Group, Kansas City, Missouri

Library of Congress Control Number: 2010922359

ISBN: 978-0-87159-345-0

Canada BN 13252 0933 RT

*This book is dedicated to all of those who, despite the difficulty, have the strength and courage to make the best wellness choices in their lives every day.*

# Contents

# Foreword

It has been several years since I joined the chorus of those encouraging Dr. Michelle Robin to write a book capturing the wisdom and practical magic she has acquired during her passionate pursuit of health and well-being. Like Dr. Abraham Maslow, who revolutionized our understanding of mental health by his radical choice to focus his study on exceptionally well people instead of only the ill, Dr. Robin has spent her two-decade medical practice focusing on how to support optimal well-being. And she has succeeded! Her study and support of what truly maximizes healthy living have led her to develop one of the leading wellness centers in the United States. She has been vigilant in her own healing, and kind and generous in providing her patients and friends (often one and the same) with an integrated approach to improving and maintaining good health.

Dr. Robin understands that we are spiritual beings having a human experience. On this journey to radiant health and freedom, we must transform our thinking, feelings, body temple, relationships and environment to establish harmony in our lives. This understanding informs the practices she suggests in this book, and these practices will transform your life.

It may seem incredible that 100 years ago, the mind-body-spirit connection was a radical and mostly unknown concept. Shortly after Unity's co-founder Myrtle Fillmore was given a terminal diagnosis and told she had only a few months to live, she heard a simple truth that would change her life and influence millions as her understanding of Truth expanded.

"You are a child of God and do not inherit sickness" was a seed idea that took root in her soul and inspired Fillmore to embark on a quest to understand the principles embodied in Jesus' healings. Her total and complete healing was realized, not by a theoretical understanding but through precious hours sitting in the silence and listening to Spirit and by a daily and consistent application of the truths she discovered. As Fillmore received more guidance, she put her new insights into practice and became willing to share what she had learned with others who sought her help.

Dr. Robin understands at a soul level the universal principles that Fillmore's dramatic healing revealed. Her own transformation has involved different aspects of her being but has been the result of a similar commitment and willingness to make the changes necessary for well-being that Fillmore's life revealed. Like Fillmore, her desire to be of service has blessed many who have come to her for help.

The ideas offered in the little book you hold in your hands have improved my life. They offer you an invitation as well as an affirmation that you deserve to be radiantly healthy and filled with joy. It contains what the Buddhists call *skillful means:* seven areas to focus on that naturally lead to your increased well-being. And the best news is that they are available to everyone. But only you can take the steps and make the changes that become a way of life. I encourage you to begin. As you read each chapter, be sure to take time to acknowledge all the aspects of your life that are working. What's right about you is more than enough to transform and heal the rest, and it is a simple but important truth that what you appreciate appreciates!

~

Remember this! The full realization of Fillmore's health took a couple of years of daily practice, but out of her efforts grew the worldwide movement called Unity. Dr. Robin's wisdom has been two decades in the making but has led to the creation of a wellness center that serves thousands of patients every year. Life has no less wonder in store for you. Truly you are a child of God, worthy of great well-being and designed for magnificence. Dare to begin the journey. What lies before you will delight and amaze you, and might even change your world for good.

I have been richly blessed by Michelle Robin's devotion to health. I pray that you will be as well.

*Rev. Mary Omwake*
*Peaceful Mind, Joyful Heart Ministries*
*Maui, Hawaii*

# Introduction

The initial inspiration for this book grew from my own life experiences, the challenges and opportunities that have made me who I am today. As I look back over my journey, I am humbled by the sustaining and healing grace of God.

I am the chief wellness officer and founder of Your Wellness Connection in Shawnee, Kansas (located in the Kansas City, Missouri, metropolitan area). In 1997, after practicing as a doctor of chiropractic medicine for five years, I began to ask myself, "Is this *all* there is to life?" I was carrying around significant unresolved pain. Like many people, I'd had a challenging upbringing. My father abandoned our family when I was very young, and he was dead by the time I was 9 years old. My stepfather suffered from alcoholism. I experienced sexual abuse. I have no memory of a time that my mother was not sick. And because we moved every couple of years when I was a child, I never had any sense of belonging.

Though outwardly I was a successful doctor and business-woman, during moments when I was completely honest with myself, I had to face the truth that I had become someone I did not respect, someone I did not even like. I knew that I could no longer live the way I had been living. I called my minister and asked for help.

My search for help and healing led me in October 1997 to the Hoffman Process, an eight-day experience that helped me identify my negative thought and belief patterns and replace them with positive ones. This was a pivotal point in my journey.

Today I continue to heal the negative patterns I learned as a child. I work to be emotionally present to myself and to all those I encounter. In spite of the pain, I know with 100 percent certainty that my soul chose my family and my life's experiences so that I could work compassionately with my clients and fall madly in love with my mission: to connect and inspire others to live well.

Currently, my own greatest challenge is being patient with myself as I seek to live congruently with the lifestyle tips and practices that I teach others. I know it is not easy to make the best wellness choice every moment. I, like you, struggle each day to eat the right food, to exercise and to think positively. I applaud you for your strength, commitment and courage. I am filled with gratitude to be able to walk beside you on this journey! For nearly two decades I have guided and supported people on their journeys toward total wellness. As my colleagues and I at Your Wellness Connection have worked intimately with thousands of people, one truth has become clear: All human beings are designed to be well. I also believe that we are whole beings—body, mind, heart and soul—and that health or disease in one area is profoundly connected to health or disease elsewhere.

Every day I meet people who truly want to feel better, to have lives and bodies that really work, to enjoy their existence and not merely "make it through another day." Simultaneously, they lament that healthy living costs a lot of money, and they are afraid that in the current economy—or even in any economy—wellness is beyond their reach.

~

# Introduction

I disagree! Wellness is attainable, and you can definitely be well on a shoestring budget. Whether people have millions or are living at the poverty level (and I've worked with those at both ends of the spectrum and everywhere in between), I have seen time and again that those who consistently practice the seven behaviors outlined in this book do very well.

I embarked upon the journey of writing this book to share these seven practices with you. I invited Rev. Roxanne Renée Grant to contribute to these concepts and share my voice as we explore these simple wellness practices. I want to inspire you to live a vibrant, well life—a life of wholeness and joy. It's both easier and harder than you think. It's easy because the concepts I share are simple and basic to life. You probably already know them, although you may not know how powerfully they affect your well-being every single day.

On the other hand, it's hard. It's hard because living well requires you to be intentional, to use your personal power to support your health, on purpose and without apology, in a culture where the majority of people around you do not practice a wellness lifestyle. Wellness is really a matter of purposeful habit, the day-in-and-day-out living of basic practices. I understand that these concepts are not exciting or sexy in and of themselves, but I contend that a truly well person is absolutely exciting and, without question, sexy and vibrant.

With this book I invite you to "act out," outside our society's norm—that is, to live differently from all of those people you know who have lives that are less than the life you want. I invite you to join me in learning, practicing and sharing a wellness lifestyle that leads to a phenomenal experience of life! It is my fervent hope and prayer (yes, I do have an agenda) that this book will inspire you to become a rebel with a cause, that your life of wholeness will spill over into the lives around you and become part of the healing energy so desperately needed on our planet.

This book is organized into seven chapters, each one made up of five parts: a series of questions to help you reflect upon how you are currently practicing one aspect of wellness; an explanation of the wellness behavior itself; stories of others who are practicing or working to incorporate into their lives this aspect of wellness; practical tips to help you as you journey forward; and an area for your notes. At the end of the book, I offer a section of resources where you can find more information on any given topic.

All personal stories shared in this book are based on the real-life experiences of those with whom I or my co-author has worked, although I have occasionally changed a name or two and a few minor details to protect their privacy. It is important to note that the exact methods used in each personal story may not work for you, nor will every tip listed at the end of the chapter be one you want to try. You must create your own path. Also, please be sure—especially if you have or develop any health concerns—that you discuss them with a medical and/or wellness professional.

There is no particular order to the concepts in this book. They do not build upon one another sequentially; rather, they are all integral pieces of a wellness lifestyle that supports vibrant health for human beings. The purpose of this book is to make people aware that a journey into wellness doesn't have to be an overwhelming undertaking. Instead, it can be done a little at a time, in whatever order makes you happy.

In addition, being well doesn't have to cost a fortune, and that's the fundamental principle upon which this book is based: wellness on a shoestring. The capacity for living a life of wellness is within all of us—we just need to resolve to do it, one tiny step at a time. And as you'll see in the chapters to come, most of these practices don't cost a cent.

Feel free to use this book any way you feel led to do so. You can work through the concepts alone or with a group to provide support and encouragement as you make lifestyle changes. You can read this book straight through from beginning to end; but if you prefer, jump right into the chapters or sections that seem most relevant to your life right now. Read parts of it now and parts in the future, or work through one concept at a time, making sure you master one wellness practice before adopting another. You can even read the habits in reverse order, starting with the seventh. It's up to you. This is your journey, and you are the most relevant expert regarding your own life. Ask yourself what you need to read right now, and then begin. If you're ready, let's do it!

Enjoy!

*Michelle Robin, D.C.*
*Chief Wellness Officer and Founder*
*Your Wellness Connection*
*Shawnee, Kansas*

# Chapter 1

# Rest, Reflect and Rejuvenate

In order to maximize your wellness, you need time to slow down, relax, repair and re-energize. You can do this by providing your mind, body and spirit with restorative activities and outlets. Before we discuss what you need and how to obtain it, take stock of how you feel and how you currently give yourself opportunities to rest, reflect and rejuvenate.

## Questions to Consider

- How much sleep do you regularly get each night? What is your usual sleep position?

- When do you usually go to bed? What is your bedtime routine?

- Do you have difficulty falling asleep? Do you wake up during the night? How often? What do you do before going back to sleep?

- When do you usually awaken? Do you awaken on your own, or do you need an alarm clock? Do you usually sleep deeply and awaken feeling refreshed?

- How do you feel most days when you get out of bed?

- Do you regularly find yourself needing stimulants (like caffeine and sugar) or stimulating activities in order to have enough energy to get through your day?

- How often do you find yourself using alcohol or other mind-altering substances to unwind?

- In the course of your normal day or week, what activities fill you with energy?

~

ᐁ If you could go anywhere right now in order to rejuvenate, where would you go? What would you do there?
   Who would be with you?

ᐁ Have you spent time outdoors in the past week?

ᐁ Do you engage in any regular spiritual practice? What is
   it?

ᐁ Are you present to the joy and wonder in your own life?
   How do you know?

---

## The Power of Rejuvenation

"A good laugh and a long sleep are the best cures in
the doctor's book."

—Irish proverb

"In every walk with nature one receives far more
than he seeks."

—John Muir

---

The first wellness practice in this book focuses on those
energizing, life-giving, enjoyable (aka "fun!") activities that
rejuvenate us. As of this moment, consider yourself under
doctor's orders to regularly pursue and practice behaviors
that leave you feeling rested, refreshed, relaxed and happy.
It's not selfish to have fun, to take a break, to vacation, to
unwind, to laugh—in fact, it's quite the opposite: Those very
things are integral to self-care.

In a society that places so much emphasis on productivity,
we often feel guilty about taking any time away from doing

the kinds of work that can be measured in concrete ways. In truth, getting regular downtime is key to productive stamina and the process of creativity, just as rest is key to the process of building physical strength. Here is the equation: *(less time at work) + (more time resting and having fun) = higher productivity!*

And yet many people continue to wear stress-related illnesses (and how many of our modern illnesses are not stress-related?) like badges of honor: "Look how committed I am to caring for my family!" or "Look how dedicated I am to this company!" We get up and show up early, stay late and go to bed later, work through lunch and dinner or eat as we drive to our next commitment, and skip our workouts and cancel play dates as though taking time for sleep and nourishment and movement and fun were optional. Then we're surprised when we get sick.

Our bodies are so perfectly designed that they will get our attention, one way or another, when we neglect their basic needs. It was an eye-opening day when I realized that most of my illnesses were not "caught"; rather, I had "earned" them—through the lifestyle choices I made day after day that depleted my strength and my immune system. Far from discouraging me, however, this knowledge gave me power: If I can live into disease, then I can live into wellness too, and so can everyone else.

## Sleep: There Is No Substitute

Rejuvenation is a key wellness practice that includes, but is certainly not limited to, the deeply restorative activity of sleep. Since sleep is so profoundly important, however, I'll address it first. I cannot think of one physical, mental, emotional or spiritual condition that cannot be supported and improved by consistent, good sleep. Each of us has the ability to experience this kind of sleep—we just have to focus on it, making sleep a priority in our busy lives.

In a 2008 lecture, Sarah J. Hon, D.O., a neurologist with Northland Neurological Associates in Kansas City, Missouri, explained that sleep is when the body repairs itself, processes information and stores it in memory so that we can be prepared for future activities. Simply stated, the brain just doesn't work without adequate sleep. When people go three or more days in a row without any sleep, they may develop symptoms that mimic psychosis, such as experiencing paranoia or hallucinations. Sleep deprivation leads to weakened immune system function; increased risk of heart disease; impaired brain function, including a decreased ability to regulate glucose, cortisol and insulin (which increases the risk of obesity and non-insulin-dependent, or type 2, diabetes); reduced brain efficiency in terms of memory, learning, creativity and problem-solving; increased accidents and errors; and a higher risk of depression and anxiety. In fact, according to Dr. Hon, people with persistent insomnia are 40 times more likely to develop depression within a year than those who sleep well.

In addition to sleep itself, the way you sleep is very important. Your sleep position has a direct impact on the ability of your nervous system to function well. Think about this: All the nerves in your body feed into the spinal cord, and information is transmitted back and forth from the brain to the billions of cells via this neurological information superhighway. The nervous system controls every single activity of the body.

How effectively can that happen if the spinal column is out of alignment?

When you sleep on your stomach, you stress your spinal cord and force it out of its natural position. Think about the kink formed in the neck area when you lie on your stomach—ouch! Sleeping with your arms over the head; with fisted hands, tense shoulders and one hip shifted; or with pillows that are too high can impair nervous system functioning and can be downright painful. It is important to position your body in a posture that supports the neck in its natural curvature and allows for an aligned spine.

Good sleep posture means sleeping on your back or on your side with a pillow between your knees. It's important to have level hips, relaxed shoulders and relaxed hands. Sleeping with your hands in an awkward position can lead to numbness, pain and even carpal tunnel syndrome.

One of my colleagues at Your Wellness Connection (YWC), Michael Brown, is a licensed naturopathic physician (N.D.). A naturopathic doctor attends four years of graduate-level education at an accredited naturopathic medicine school and is educated in all the same basic sciences as a medical doctor (M.D.), but also studies holistic and nontoxic therapies with a strong emphasis on preventing disease and optimizing wellness. Dr. Brown notes, "Every time a patient comes in, one of the first things I ask is how he or she is sleeping. If you're having trouble going to sleep or staying asleep, something systemically is going on. If you're not sleeping, something is out of balance."

He points out that when and how sleep is occurring (or not occurring, as the case may be) are powerful clues to underlying conditions. For example, it's very common for menopausal women who are estrogen-deficient to awaken between 2 and 3 a.m. night after night. Likewise, if you awaken fatigued or completely exhausted, day after day, no matter how much sleep you get, you could have adrenal issues. If you have a glass of wine to unwind or a late-night snack within an hour or two of bed, don't be surprised if you wake up in the middle of the night or toss and turn. Your blood sugar has shifted while you were sleeping, which can disturb your ability to rest and reach a deeper level of sleep.

It's important to listen to the message your body is sending you through your own sleep patterns. Anytime you are not feeling fully well, pay attention to how you are sleeping and make notes. When you visit a wellness professional, bring along those notes and discuss them in detail; they will provide valuable data for guiding you toward wellness.

Although it's true that age, diet and general health affect the amount of sleep each of us needs and normal sleep patterns do vary from person to person, a general rule is that most of us need seven to nine hours of restful sleep every night. As I stated earlier, almost all the body's activities of significant repair and detoxification occur while we sleep. Deep sleep increases melatonin, which promotes immune system function, protects us from viruses, and has phenomenal anti-cancer properties. Deep sleep also increases human growth hormone, which plays an integral role in maintaining optimal body weight and helps us feel more youthful and energized.

It's probably no surprise to you that sleep deprivation triggers a vicious circle. Fatigue causes us to crave foods that are not good for us—such as foods high in caffeine, carbohydrates and sugar—or seek stimulating activities. As a result, we sleep less and grow more sleep-deprived. When we don't sleep, the immune system becomes less and less effective, unable to protect us. Thus we begin a downward spiral into disease. We become less and less able to think clearly, as well as accident-prone and irritable. Our health, relationships and productivity all deteriorate.

But here's the good news: When we reverse the process and get regular, restful sleep, everything begins to work better! Mental focus and concentration sharpen, mood lifts, irritability decreases, and energy and motivation increase. In addition, our ability to work out, to eat well and to relate in positive ways with loved ones, friends, co-workers and people in general is significantly enhanced. All of this benefit comes from regular, restful sleep … something we all enjoy anyway! How great is that?

As a practice, even if just occasional, naps can be very helpful. Some people benefit from a 10- to 15-minute "power nap," while others need up to an hour to feel refreshed. If you find yourself needing naps each day that are several hours long, however, you probably are not getting adequate rest during the night. Listen to your body and notice the way you feel after a nap, and you'll learn what works for you.

## Restfulness Beyond Sleep

In addition to sound sleep, other activities are powerfully rejuvenating and important in maintaining wellness. The custom in some countries of a siesta—a time each day when activities stop so that people can rest for a few hours—is a very healthy practice. We can't all move abroad, but we can apply some of that wisdom to our everyday lives. Consider ways for you to take time out from your work each day and do something rejuvenating, like 10 to 15 minutes of yoga, meditating, listening to music you like, or walking outdoors to experience nature and sunshine. For many of us, direct contact with another living being—interaction with a good friend, laughing with your children or even playing with a pet—is most restorative. Reaching out and feeling connected via social-networking outlets, like Facebook or MySpace—in moderation—can also make for a nice break in your day and refresh your focus.

One of the most rejuvenating activities you can participate in for wellness is some form of regular spiritual practice during which you are present in the moment. It could be praying, chanting, meditating, gardening, hiking, even drinking a cup of coffee ritualistically every morning—anything you do in which you stay in the moment. The key is not to think but simply to be—to be present to whatever is happening and detach from your ego mind.

Frustration occurs when our ego mind says, "The world isn't the way I think it should be!" This allows for no trust in a higher power, no faith in a bigger plan than what can currently be seen or comprehended with our limited understanding. Anytime you feel yourself becoming frustrated, ask yourself, "What is happening here that I think should be different? Should it really be different, or am I frustrated because I am trying to control something, insisting on my way?" Releasing the need to control can immediately shift our frustration to a more relaxed state, allowing us to function in better ways. And if indeed something does need to be changed, we are better able to bring about that change from a place of calm thinking than a place of frustration.

In the present *moment*, much of the time, everything is perfect. If we can cease to worry over future possibilities and can stop rehashing past experiences, choosing to focus solely on right here and right now, we usually find that we have everything we need at that moment. How often are we really in life-threatening situations? Almost never! But the ego mind creates them, and we spend countless hours in fight-or-flight response to threats that have already passed or have not yet materialized.

Spiritual practice that keeps us in the present allows us to detach from the ego mind, to watch ourselves and our reactions without judgment, and to offer ourselves compassion. We can begin to see that the ego mind allows us to function in the world, but it is not the self. With intention and practice, we get better and better at detaching from the ego mind and operating out of spirit, the true self. This is profoundly rejuvenating and supports vibrant wellness.

Another deeply rejuvenating activity that supports wellness is the regular experience of nature. In modern daily life, we are bombarded with myriad energy frequencies. The vibrations from radio, television, computers, cell phones and countless other electronic devices affect us in ways that we don't yet entirely comprehend. What we do understand is that we are energy beings. Our bodies are matter, which is simply energy vibrating very slowly, and energy vibrations from other sources can affect us on many levels.

When we experience nature, we are as close as we can get to pure Christ Presence or Consciousness or God or whatever you may call this phenomenon/power. Being in the natural world is profoundly healing for people; just a walk in the woods behind your house or a walk through the nearest neighborhood park is healing. It is imperative for wellness that you regularly spend time in nature, to be supported by the natural vibrations of living things.

Spending time outside to reconnect with nature affects your wellness another way: It gives you the benefit of the vitamin D your body needs and can absorb in as little as 15 minutes outdoors. Studies show that Americans are significantly deficient in this vitamin, which plays an important role in the intestines' absorption of calcium and phosphorus. Calcium, as you know, is critical to keeping bones strong throughout growth and aging. Vitamin D can even contribute to proper thyroid and kidney functions. (You'll learn more about how vitamin D contributes to wellness in Chapter 6.)

When you spend time in nature, whether it is to exercise or just to enjoy the outdoors, get in touch with all of your senses. Ask yourself, "What do I smell? What do I hear? What can I reach out and touch? How does it feel? What is the texture and temperature? What do I see? What can I taste (like salt water or rain)?" Be aware through all of your senses. Take a moment to be in thanksgiving, asking, "What am I grateful for in this moment?"

Here's another rejuvenating activity that supports wellness: Spend regular time doing things you love to do! Decide which activities bring you life, activities during which you have no sense of time passing because you are so engaged, activities after which you feel happier and more sane, rested, energized and alive. Then plan time each day, week, month and year to do those things.

It's also important to spend time having fun with your family and friends. Humans are social beings; we need regular interaction with others in order to be well. Planning such time is especially important for people who live or work alone, because negative, obsessive, stress-inducing thinking (also called ruminating) seems to occur most often when we are alone and idle. Good friendships and consistent social support can help heal conditions like depression and social anxiety.

I recently took up cycling. I found out it is a lot more fun and I am a lot more apt to do it when I go on a ride with friends. I also regularly get together with a group of friends to play cards, laugh and have fun. It is important to note that I am not just talking about spending time with people. You do that when you serve on a nonprofit board or the PTA. While I certainly believe that it is good for the soul to be engaged in the community, these activities usually come with "to-dos." I want you to take time to have fun for the sake of fun!

Renowned motivational speaker and self-help author Wayne W. Dyer, Ph.D., in his book *The Power of Intention*[1], discusses a study demonstrating that random acts of kindness, with no credit going to those carrying out the acts, are a powerful wellness practice. Among those on the receiving end, immune system parameters, including serotonin levels (the "feel good" brain chemicals), showed statistically significant increases. But it turns out that those who performed the random acts of kindness received the same immune system boosts. Even more amazing, the physiological rewards extended to people who had only witnessed these actions! Our acts of kindness—even simply offering a smile or a compliment to another human being—are powerfully positive enhancers for physiological, mental, spiritual and emotional wellness.

Another way to rejuvenate our bodies is by drinking adequate amounts of water (more about this in Chapter 7) and taking key supplements. An easy way to know how much water to drink is to divide your body weight in pounds by two. Take the resulting number and let it represent the number of ounces of water you should consume daily. For example, if you weigh 140 pounds, a daily consumption of 70 ounces of fresh water is indicated. Adequate water consumption is important no matter what age you are. Also consider taking a multivitamin and fish-oil supplements every day.

Finally, don't stress yourself out over this process! Remember that wellness is an individual journey, and it's not all or nothing. You can commit to health and wellness five days each week, then take a break for two days, and you'll still make excellent progress. Allow yourself to take baby steps in which you set yourself up to succeed; define your success in small, measurable goals that you move toward at a rate that works for you and for your life.

Don't be overwhelmed by this book or *any* book. Don't be overwhelmed by thoughts of what you need to do to improve your well-being. If you like, randomly open this book and work on whatever's on that page for a day, a week, two weeks, a month—whatever time you need to fully incorporate the new habit into your life. Do what works for *you*.

## Personal Stories

Patti Phillips is a friend and client who came to me eight years ago with a rare autoimmune disorder. She was taking steroids, autoimmune suppressants and other pharmaceutical drugs that were helping her somewhat, or at least managing her symptoms, but as she said to me, "In my case, I intuitively know that Western medicine is not the long-term way to go."

We began to work together, using surveys she completed about her life and experience, X-rays, blood work and the wisdom of a variety of wellness practitioners to guide us. Patti consulted with nutrition experts, saw an acupuncturist, received chiropractic adjustments and attended seminars. She learned to advocate for her own wellness and to make lifestyle choices that supported her body's phenomenal capacity for healing.

One of the first and most important changes Patti agreed to make was to commit to getting between eight and eight-and-a-half hours of sleep every night. The impact was profound—so much so that years later, she remains dedicated to getting good sleep. For her, it's nonnegotiable.

As her health improved, Patti felt empowered to make more lifestyle changes, and step by step she continued her journey of wellness. After using no medication for a year and a half, she did have a flareup of her disease. She had one last infusion of a drug but was undeterred, intending it to be her last. It was. Patti says that because her overall health was so much better than before, this infusion worked quickly to handle the last remnants of her disease. To this day, Patti is off all drugs for her condition. Miraculous? Perhaps. Or maybe simply a product of the wellness lifestyle to which Patti has committed—a lifestyle to which we can all commit.

Patti will tell you that we all need to make conscious choices to take good care of the vessels in which our spirits dwell. She knows that we cannot take health for granted, a lesson that her body eloquently, if painfully, taught her. When sharing her story with others, Patti proclaims that life is about habits and behaviors: Change your habits, change your life! It really *can* be that simple.

Sleep is such a core wellness practice that after one client recovered from a particularly severe depression, she told me that her psychiatrist warned, "For the rest of your life, no matter what, do not, under any circumstances, allow yourself to become sleep-deprived!" Any person who has lived with a mood disorder is acutely aware of how even one night's poor sleep can affect thinking, mood and the ability to respond to life's daily frustrations with patience and poise. In fact, my clients have related stories to me of their children, on a day when Mom or Dad was particularly irritable, asking, "Did you not sleep well last night?" If our children can assimilate these lessons in their own lives, there will be more and more wellness in our world!

Another wellness practice that supports healing is the reflective act of giving thanks. According to my YWC colleague Amanda Toney, D.C., "Those who have, recognize and feel gratitude heal faster." She has noticed this daily in her practice as a chiropractor. Dr. Toney shared the story of two clients with the same physical problem. One client—we'll call her Cindi Collins—is in better physical health overall and thus might be expected to heal more quickly than another client we'll refer to as Nancy Kotter. Cindi's attitude, however, is skeptical, dissatisfied, resentful and closed. Nancy, on the other hand, has an attitude of openness and acceptance. She is engaged in the process of healing and is able to express gratitude for even seemingly small graces: the beauty around her, the attention of a compassionate doctor, any positive encounter in her day, the possibility of learning something from her experience.

Although both clients have an identical treatment plan, after numerous treatments, Cindi has shown no change, while Nancy is healing. Dr. Toney points out that when the body has too much energy tied up in maintaining negative emotions, such as resentment or anger, energy is not free to support healing and to sustain wellness.

Noah Webster's 1828 dictionary defines the state of being content this way: "Rest or quietness of the mind in the present condition; satisfaction which holds the mind in peace, restraining complaint, opposition or further desire, and often implying a moderate degree of happiness." Though it may seem backward, being content where we are right now is the starting point from which we move toward greater wellness. Our acceptance of the present situation, without judgment or bitterness or anger, allows every cell in our bodies to focus energy on the situation at hand. Anger and bitterness keep us stuck in the past; judgment shames and imprisons us. Acceptance and gratitude, however, connect us to that part of ourselves that trusts the universe and expects good, unleashing the power of faith … a power that heals disease and sustains wellness.

## Practical Tips for Your Journey

Take some time for reflection as you practice the following exercises:

1. As you awaken for the day, in that peaceful space between sleeping and being fully alert, let the first words that you breathe out be "thank you." Say the phrase as many times as you desire. You may wish to offer thanks for specific things, picturing them in your mind as you do, but it is not necessary. Simply begin your conscious day with the breath prayer of "thank you."

2. Take some time to pay attention—really pay attention—to what you see around you. Choose something and look at it as if this were the very first time you've ever seen it. Let go of anything you think you know about this object or person or experience and allow your senses to bring you information. Allow yourself to get caught up in the wonder, the miracle that you are observing. Feel your body's response. Breathe deeply. Allow yourself to stand in awe.

3. Find something beautiful and focus on it. Allow yourself to take in the beauty you see; allow the beauty to fill you. Imagine this beauty as energy, and source yourself from it, as though it were recharging your internal battery. When you feel "full," imagine sending some of this beauty/energy to someone else who needs it. Imagine the beauty/energy refilling you as you share it with someone else. Give thanks for the beauty around you and the way you are able to respond to beauty.

4. Think of a person or an activity that makes you laugh. It could be a friend or a group of friends, a book, a television show or a movie—anything that makes you laugh

deeply, from your gut. Schedule a time to be with your friend or friends or to participate in those activities within the next five days. Keep your appointment with fun as though it were an urgent priority, absolutely integral to your health. It is not frivolous; it is powerfully healing. Just do it!

5. Set a timer for a short length of time, say one minute. Sit in silence with your own thoughts. Observe them, and do not judge them or try to control them in any way. Do not distract yourself with music or any activity. Be still and simply breathe. If you notice yourself thinking or feeling something unpleasant, get some distance by saying, "Isn't that interesting, how I [*fill in the blank with whatever you are thinking or feeling*]?" Watch your mind as though you were a scientist; get to know how it works. As you get better at this practice, set the timer for longer and longer periods of time. What do you learn about yourself as you get better at being present with your own soul?

6. Play the "I love …" game with a friend or loved one. You simply take turns remembering the little things that make you happy and feel relaxed. This exercise can be rejuvenating in and of itself. For instance, I love to luxuriate in a hot bath with a magazine at the end of a long day. I love crawling into clean sheets fresh from the dryer. I love the smell of neighbors' fireplaces going in the fall. I love baking cookies with the kids. I love playing golf. I love that feeling when I really don't "have to" do anything. You get the idea.

Set yourself up for great sleep by practicing good sleep hygiene:

1. Invest in a good mattress, excellent pillows that support your neck in a natural alignment and high-quality bed linens—the best you can afford without going into debt.

2. Notice the position in which you usually sleep. Train yourself to sleep on your back, with a pillow under your knees if needed; or on your side, with a pillow between your knees. Practice relaxing your neck, shoulders, arms and hands. Be sure not to sleep with your arms over your head.

3. Decide when you need to be up each morning; subtract seven to nine hours, depending on your personal requirement; and plan this as your optimum bedtime. About an hour-and-a-half before this time, turn down the lights and the temperature and turn off your computer to signal your brain to begin getting you ready for sleep. About 15 to 30 minutes before bedtime, start your slowdown routine, which includes taking care of personal hygiene and doing relaxation practices like meditation or prayer. Consider taking a hot shower or bath to soothe the body and wash away the energy of the day.

4. Plan to get up the same time every day, including weekends, to support your natural sleeping rhythms.

5. Wear loose, comfortable clothing to bed.

6. Keep the TV and computer out of the bedroom, and use the bed for sleeping and sensual activities only!

⁓

7. Add white noise such as a fan, relaxing sounds or music to drown out any distracting noises that could keep you awake.

8. For maximum natural relaxation, observe the following: no vigorous exercise 1.5 hours before bed, no alcohol or nicotine 1.5 hours before bed, no caffeine three hours before bed, and no eating three hours before bed.

9. Make sure you are supporting your body's ability to rest by dealing with any allergies and treating any pain you may have.

10. If you cannot fall asleep within 15 to 20 minutes, stop trying. Get out of bed and do something else. If your mind is full, write your thoughts down on paper, emptying your mind so you can relax. Try a short walk, a yoga pose or other light activity. When you find yourself feeling sleepy, go back to bed.

## Your Space

Use this page to make notes and write your thoughts on resting, reflecting and rejuvenating.

# Chapter 2

# Breathe Deeply

Breath is looked upon as life, as spirit, throughout world cultures. Breath has both physiological and emotional connections. Breathing is both reactionary and proactive. Your breathing will respond to your physical or emotional circumstances; you can also control your breathing to affect your physical and emotional responses. Breath is energizing, cleansing and restorative—physically, emotionally and even spiritually. Before I discuss how interwoven breath is into the well-being of your mind-body-spirit, take a moment to assess your awareness of your own well-being and the quality of your breathing.

## Questions to Consider

- Do you fight chronic illness or have other symptoms of a weakened immune system?
- Are you sensitive to toxins in the air, such as smoke, perfume, household cleaners and/or lawn chemicals?
- Are you aware of your breathing?
- When you breathe, do you feel your ribs expand?
- Do you notice when your breath speeds up or slows down?
- Do you find yourself holding your breath?
- Do you find yourself sighing a lot?
- Do you snore?
- Are you ever short of breath?

- Do you experience episodes of panic?

- Do you practice a time of conscious breathing each day? If not daily, how often? For what period of time do you practice conscious breathing?

- Are you aware of others' breathing and the effect it has on your own?

- When you are with others, can you regulate your breathing in ways that enable or support a calm response from those around you?

---

## The Power of Breathing

"Stress is basically a disconnection from the earth, a forgetting of the breath. Stress is an ignorant state. It believes that everything is an emergency. Nothing is that important."

—Natalie Goldberg

"Breathe. Let go. And remind yourself that this very moment is the only one you know you have for sure."

—Oprah Winfrey

---

Think about the last time you were looking forward to something really exciting. Did your breathing speed up? Could you feel your heart in your chest? Did you gasp in surprise or delight? Did the moment quite literally take your breath away?

Now think about the last time you felt anxious about something, or afraid. Did your breathing speed up? Could you feel your heart in your chest? Did you gasp in shock, horror or outrage? Did the moment lock up your muscles, causing you to hold yourself so tightly that even your breathing ceased?

Good or bad, high or low, our emotions are intimately connected to our breathing. We reveal our inner state by the way we breathe. Every feeling, every experience we have affects our breathing. And the reverse is also true: The way we breathe affects our experiences and the way we process our emotions.

Each week I deal with people in some kind of crisis. One of the first and most important things I do is help them regulate their breathing so that it is deep and even. This act alone has a powerfully calming effect and enables them to think more clearly, to process necessary information and to make good decisions.

Breathing well is arguably the most important thing you can do for your health. Without breath, there is no life at all. It is for this reason that human beings from earliest times have connected the life force within to the breath. Before the advent of machines that register precisely when the brain dies, the moment of death was the moment one stopped breathing.

In religious belief systems such as Judaism, Christianity and Islam, the breath of God is a powerful, life-giving force. We have images of God forming humans by hand and breathing into their lungs to impart life. We are inspired by religious scriptures and writings, including those of St. Paul, that use words such as the Greek term *theopneustos*, which means "God-breathed" or "breathed out by God." And in the spiritual practices of many cultures, time periods and lands, we see focused breathing used as a tool to bring one into a state of meditation—that calm, clear, focused state of alpha brain wave patterns that is so beneficial to our health and well-being.

The great thing is, breathing is a wellness practice that is absolutely free! You can practice intentional deep breathing anywhere and anytime. Deep breathing affects every system of the body in positive ways. The next section, which is based on ideas from exercise physiologist Ciardha Carey, examines the physiological process of breathing and its powerful effects on well-being.

## The Mechanics of Breath

"We are supposed to be in a relaxed state naturally. We are supposed to take forays into the flight-or-fight response, but we're not supposed to stay there!"

—Ciardha Carey

Carey, who was interviewed for this book, has spent years studying the applied system of breath mechanics, which presents an understanding of what breathing does and every system it affects. We can look at breathing as the hub of a wheel: Our physical, energetic, emotional and mental aspects all connect through breathing, much as spokes of a wheel connect at the center hub. By moving our breath deep into the body—meaning deep breathing that is slow and relaxed and fully engages the diaphragm (the muscle running horizontally below the lungs) and completely expands the intercostal (rib) muscles—we affect each of those aspects simultaneously.

The power of conscious breathing is inherent in the body's design. All you have to do is reawaken your dormant intelligence, your dormant understanding of conscious breathing, and through practice you can begin breathing at your own most efficient rate. It doesn't matter if you have breathed poorly for years. Once you start to breathe deeply and well, your entire system is reactivated according to original design and immediately begins to bring you benefits.

It's easy to see this process at work when you are under stress. The muscles of respiration tend to be the first to respond to negative emotions; there is always a response of tension that occurs at the edges of the range of motion. This means that when you are worried, anxious, angry or afraid, you stop breathing fully in and out. You decrease your range of breathing motion; you lock down. As your system gets less oxygen, you are less able to sustain a state of well-being on all levels.

This is actually a defense mechanism, because less breath equals less feeling. This is fine if you need to focus on survival by, let's say, fleeing a tiger. In the moment of attack, being able to process how you feel about being attacked is not of primary importance. In fact, it could be rather distracting and could get you eaten! But that kind of "don't feel" defense mechanism is designed to be a very, very short-term situation. In our world, we tend to get stuck in our stress response, and this has long-term negative effects on health. In a state of perpetual stress, we never find our way to feeling relaxed.

What happens physiologically when you don't breathe deeply is an imbalance of gases in the body. The greater amount of carbon dioxide has a numbing effect. How? Carbon is one of the most insulating properties in the universe; it blocks electrical transfer so that the tissues become less electrically conductive. When you breathe deeply for, say, 30 minutes, there is a cascade effect in which you release carbon dioxide and bring in oxygen, which allows the neurons to conduct more impulses—tiny electrical signals—in the nervous system. The system can rebalance and get to work, moving out lactic acid, stimulating the brain's vagus nerve (which puts you into an alpha brain wave state of calm awareness) and engaging the parasympathetic (or relaxation) nervous system response.

Another phenomenal benefit of deep breathing is the processing of stuck emotions. For every emotion you don't fully express and feel, there are chemicals called neuropeptides that have bonded to receptor sites in the body. There they sit, waiting to fire as the emotion is processed and released. If they are not processed, layer upon layer can build up, stuck there for an indeterminate amount of time as stored emotional tension.

Stretching out the muscles of respiration leads to the release of that stored tension. It is not uncommon for this to happen during a massage as you allow yourself to breathe deeply and relax. You may find yourself crying or releasing emotions of which you were not aware. What is happening is that the neuropeptides are finally getting enough oxygen, enabling them to fire and thus be released and moved out of the body. As you breathe deeply, you become aware of the tension, and you can choose either to continue processing it or to stop breathing so deeply. But if you choose not to process your tension, you make it impossible for the body to enter a state of deep relaxation.

By consciously and regularly practicing breathing through all the ranges of motion of the diaphragm and intercostal muscles, you will come into contact with any tension or pain you are manifesting physiologically that resulted from a negative emotional issue. This issue will always be related to a belief of some kind that you hold. Find the belief causing the pain, shift the belief causing the pain and alleviate the pain. Thus, conscious use of breathing becomes a very useful tool for understanding yourself, unraveling the mystery of your own life and contemplating, "Why don't I have more harmony, peace and balance?" Your breathing can guide you to resolve and shift beliefs and behaviors that are not working in your life. It becomes a system of self-referential feedback in which you watch and learn about every aspect of yourself.

## Breathing and Meditation

"Meditation is the tongue of the soul and the language of our spirit."

—Jeremy Taylor

What I've been describing is an ancient teaching about the importance of breathing, and it leads us to consider the practice of meditation. Breathing is the first, most effective gateway to one's ability to meditate. The heart, which lies right above the diaphragm in your body, will adjust itself to the rate of your breathing. Thus, when you breathe deeply and slowly, the cardiovascular system slows down into greater relaxation. As you breathe consciously, you unravel stuck emotions. You breathe; they surface. You express them; they leave. As you develop your breathing more and more, your body learns to dwell in this relaxed state.

Jill Tupper, a life coach and energy practitioner at YWC, says that when you begin to still yourself through breathing exercises or meditation, it will take some time for the static of your mind and emotions to truly settle down. She compares it to a snow globe that you shake up: You may have set the globe down, but "snow" swirls around, floats and drifts for a while before it finally settles and the waters are still. Thoughts of day-to-day busyness and any emotions you may stir up when you begin breathing exercises can take a little while to fully release, settle and calm, but you will eventually reach that state of deep relaxation.

Breathing is one of the most physiologically centralized points of your experience of living. You can only do without it for a matter of minutes! Breathing well affects all of your systems. It influences digestion. It raises your sensitivity to toxins in your environment. It makes you more aware of the emotions around you. Breath rates are contagious, in a way. In any given situation, panic can be shared. So can anger, but so can peace. By being aware of your breath and the way it changes in response to a particular person or situation, you have guidance about what you need for your own self-care.

Breathing deeply keeps you in *this* moment. Awareness of your breathing moves you deeper and deeper into dwelling in the present and thus allows you a richer experience and understanding of life. Even 10 minutes of breathing deeply and continuously (this means no pauses between breathing in and out) through the full range of motion of your muscles of respiration has a great impact on your physiology and emotional state. Breathing well predisposes you to radiant health!

Unity minister Patricia Bass shares her thoughts with us: "Spirit and breath are inextricably linked. The word *spirit* comes from a root that means 'breath.' Buddhists have understood this for millennia. Their beautiful teachings on mindfulness always begin with the breath—breathing in, breathing out, silent inward chanting. This is the essential Buddhist prayer. It is so powerful because when you bring your attention to the breath, it brings you to the present moment. The present moment is your point of power. The present moment is also the only place you can touch the Divine in you. You can't experience God tomorrow or yesterday, only now."

---

### Mindful Breath

"Breath is the bridge which connects life to consciousness, which unites your body to your thoughts."

—Thich Nhat Hanh

---

Thich Nhat Hanh, renowned Buddhist teacher, peace activist and author, further informs our views on breath and its connection to life and God. The most fundamental lesson he teaches in breath is awareness.[1] We must be quiet, breathe in and *know* it, feel it; breathe out and *know* it, feel it. As you concentrate on your breath, feeling and experiencing it, you stop thinking about everything else going on in your life. You are sharply focused on your body, not on other things in your life today or your past or future—just your body in this moment. This reconnects the body and mind.

The act of breathing, part of the autonomic nervous system (explored further in Chapter 3), is a function you don't normally have to think about. But by making breathing conscious, you can create oneness of body and mind. Breath is life. Each moment you breathe is a moment you are alive. Concentrating on your breath helps you become more aware of being in the present moment, not just while doing the breathing exercises but during other life experiences. This is mindfulness: to be available to yourself, others and God. Nature is only in the present. If you spend time dwelling on the past or concentrating on the future, you will miss life! Nhat Hanh also teaches us that it is only through this mindfulness that we can enter the kingdom of God, or heaven.

Breathing through your core gives you strength and stability. If you feel agitated, upset or vulnerable, you lack the solid foundation of stability. Feeling overwhelmed by emotion or illness makes you vulnerable. Sit with your body centered, back straight. As you breathe in and out, say, "I am stable. I am solid." Nhat Hanh asks us to consider a tree. The top of the tree is not solid; it sways in the wind and is vulnerable. The trunk, however, is firmly rooted and solid. You are like that: Your emotions and heart are at the top and can sway. But your abdomen, the core of your body, the trunk, is strong. Follow the movement of your abdomen as you breathe deeply; you will move from being vulnerable in your emotions to solid in your breath. You will remember that controlling your breath can be calming and can put you in control of your responses and even affect the emotional levels of those around you.

When you're working on incorporating mindful breathing into your life, always remember that it begins with, in Nhat Hanh's words, "the present moment, this wonderful moment." Such breathing helps you realize that you are alive. Know it, because it is a miracle! You can practice breathing anytime, anywhere—on a bus, in the kitchen, while walking, sitting at the airport or waiting in the car for your children to get out of school. Practice coordinating your breathing with your footsteps. Your lungs will tell you how many footsteps they want. Follow the beat of your lungs. Say yes and thanks to life, the earth and God!

Mindful living leaves no regrets. The energy you gain through mindfulness—the opposite of forgetfulness—can heal and transform your mind, body and spirit. This is critical to accomplishing your wellness goals. How many times have you intended to change your lifestyle for wellness and quickly found yourself easily slipping back into old habits? It is particularly difficult with all the responsibilities and projects we take on in our work and home lives. All the "to-dos" in our lives can crowd us, create static. Mindful breathing and meditation create space for the movement and freedom we crave and need in our lives for well-being. Taking time for such breathing will consistently help you tune in to your body and spirit, connect you with your intent, and keep you moving toward your goals.

Remember that breathing is automatic. It is effortless, something you don't have to think about in order for it to be in you, filling you up, giving you life; it just is. God, or spirit, is like that. Just like breath, God is always there, effortlessly filling you up with life, giving you the mind-body-spirit resources you need for well-being.

## Personal Stories

Ronda Snyder is a client who began practicing restorative yoga after a surgery to help with flexibility and because she was told it could have a positive effect on her high blood pressure. Because Ronda did not feel physical discomfort during her sessions, she was surprised that she quietly cried her way through the first three. Huge emotions surfaced as she stretched and focused on breathing deeply through the poses, guided by her instructor. Given what we know of the way in which deep breathing helps us release stored emotions, it is not surprising at all that Ronda had this powerful experience as she began her new practice of yoga.

Another client, the previously mentioned Patti Phillips, has had a profound healing response to breath work. A television sportscaster for women's basketball, Patti had a disease that affected her vocal cords and caused her to lose her voice when she was too tired or under too much stress. As you can imagine, this was a problem for someone who makes a living speaking on TV. When her disease flared up, she would rush to the ear, nose and throat specialist and get steroids and other medications that made it possible for her to (barely) talk. In desperation, Patti went to see a medical doctor at a large research hospital who specialized in the treatment of vocal cords. He told her that the damage was severe and that the only way she could possibly heal was by not speaking at all for two to four weeks, and even then there were no guarantees. This was not an option for her at that time.

Patti began to rest her voice when she could. She worked with a spiritual and personal coach named Sonia Choquette, who encouraged her to consider the ways she had "lost her voice" in her life and work. Through Choquette she met Mark Stanton Welch, a musician and educator whose CDs taught Patti a specific type of guided breath work. First she did exercises that helped her become conscious of her breath. Then she practiced a kind of cleansing breathing. This process took 13 minutes a day, and Patti would do it in the car during her drive to work.

Patti's body and voice healed. She has continued her practice of daily breath work for the past four years. Her disease has not recurred, and her health is very good. It seems strange to the Western mind, with our medical paradigm of cutting and medicating, that something as basic as deep, full, intentional breathing can work a seeming miracle, but we see again and again that, given the support it needs, the body can heal itself.

## Practical Tips for Your Journey

The following suggestions for intentional breath work come from exercise-physiologist Carey; YWC life coach and energy practitioner Tupper; and YWC yoga instructors:

1. Master the basic deep breath work. Because inhalation stimulates oxygen diffusion and exhalation stimulates carbon dioxide release, your basic breathing exercise will keep the inhalation and exhalation in balance. Breathe in

deeply, expanding your diaphragm fully (your tummy will push out) and expanding your intercostal muscles (you can feel them stretch wider). Make your inhalation last three seconds. Then breathe out deeply, pushing the air all the way out (your diaphragm will squeeze upward, toward your heart, and your intercostal muscles will pull together). Make your exhalation last three seconds. Then begin again, with no pause between breaths. Hold your hands over your lower abdomen to feel the rise and fall of your belly. When you're practicing deep breathing, it can be helpful to visualize the exhalation as starting from the center of your brow and washing down over your body like a waterfall. Visualize the exhalation as the emotions or negative energy you need to release.

2. Train your body to work aerobically—not having to move into anaerobic activity—by developing your breathing to a high degree. Practice accelerated breathing by breathing fully and deeply, using all the respiratory muscles, at a fast yet even rate for 10 minutes twice a day. This will super-load your body with oxygen, helping metabolize body fat back into usable blood sugar and into bioelectrical current. (By doing this, Carey lost 6 percent of his body fat in three months.)

3. To release plenty of carbon dioxide, and also to blow off steam (meaning, this is good to do when you are stressed, angry or anxious), make your inhalation significantly shorter than your exhalation. You can do it slowly, say by inhaling for a three-count and exhaling for a 12-count. You can also do it quickly, inhaling for a quick one-count and exhaling for a two-count, all through your nose, and then, in a movement sometimes called Breath of Fire, pushing

hard on the exhalation with your diaphragm. If you're practicing Breath of Fire, begin with 10 breaths, then increase over time. Be careful not to hyperventilate. And be sure to have some tissue handy, because this one really cleans out your nose too!

4. If you want to focus on stillness, make the pauses between your inhalations and exhalations last the same amount of time as your inhalations and exhalations. So you would count, for example, inhale-2-3, pause-2-3, exhale-2-3, pause-2-3. Try to cycle more and more slowly. What surfaces emotionally for you in the times of no breath, the times of silence?

5. For an isometric breathing exercise, try holding your diaphragm and intercostal muscles open while you breathe both in and out. Sustain this kind of breathing for approximately three minutes to start (do it while singing to a single song on the radio), and then work up to 10 minutes (or while you sing along with three songs) several times a day. If you are a vocalist, you will be familiar with this type of breathing.

6. Try a balancing breathing exercise with alternate nostril breathing. If you are feeling scattered or exhausted, you may benefit from the clarifying balance of alternate nostril breathing. With your eyes closed and while sitting or lying in a comfortable position that supports your back and legs, block the right nostril with your thumb and breathe in deeply through the left nostril. Block the left nostril and exhale from the right. Keeping the left nostril blocked, inhale on the right; block the right and go back to the left for the exhalation. Continue alternating nostrils for a few minutes according to your comfort level.

## Your Space

Use this page to make notes and write your own reflections on breathing deeply.

_____

_____

_____

_____

_____

_____

_____

_____

_____

_____

_____

_____

_____

_____

# Chapter 3

# Move Your Body

The body is designed to move. Movement not only lets you live your life the way you want but also triggers physiological and psychological responses that improve the well-being of your mind-body-spirit in many ways. You have muscles, joints, bones and a nervous system that allow this movement. As much as they need action to stay healthy, they also need care and maintenance. Before we get started, have you considered how you move your body?

## Questions to Consider

- Do you exercise some way, every day?
- When you select a parking space, do you choose the closest space to the door or do you choose a space far from the door? When you have a choice, do you take the stairs or the elevator or escalator?
- Do you use a pedometer? How many steps do you average each day?
- How much television do you watch each day?
- Outside of work, how much time do you sit in front of a computer each day?
- Do you utilize a timer at your computer and take a break every 45 minutes to get up and move?
- Do you practice good spinal hygiene? Do you regularly have chiropractic checkups and adjustments?

- Do you stretch or practice yoga daily? Do you practice regular spine-lengthening exercises?

- Do you engage in aerobic activity for at least 30 minutes, four times each week (which increases your heart rate to 70 to 80 percent of its maximum capacity)?

- Do you check your heart rate, or pulse, during your workouts?

- Do you engage in any regular strength-training activities?

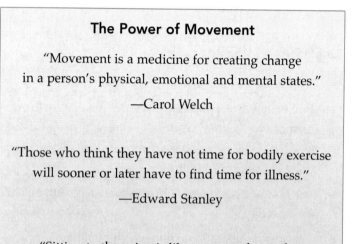

**The Power of Movement**

"Movement is a medicine for creating change
in a person's physical, emotional and mental states."
—Carol Welch

"Those who think they have not time for bodily exercise
will sooner or later have to find time for illness."
—Edward Stanley

"Sitting to the spine is like sugar to the teeth."
—Dr. James L. Chestnut

Most of the emphasis on movement in our society has to do with aerobic exercise and how important it is for cardio-vascular health. Or we hear about strength training and how critical it is for weight management and strong bones. This is all true, and we will address both aerobic exercise and strength training in this chapter, but I also want you to think about movement in a broader, more profound sense. Specifically, I want you to think about it not only as powerfully effective stress relief but also in terms of your whole-body wellness and the health of your nervous system specifically. If your nervous system cannot move messages from your brain to your organs and muscles, your body will not be able to function optimally.

How does movement affect whole-body wellness and relieve stress? I asked my YWC colleague Rafael Durán, who has been teaching Iyengar yoga for the past 16 years, for his insights. (A form of hatha yoga, Iyengar yoga is known for its use of props such as belts, blocks and bolsters. It focuses on the structural alignment of the body, building strength, balance and flexibility through the practice of postures or poses.) Not only is Durán a teacher, but he also has his own story of healing. As a teen, he had a gymnastic accident that resulted in broken vertebrae. By the time he was in his 30s, he was in constant pain, and nothing could relieve it. He decided to start chiropractic treatment (I'll explain how this works later in the chapter) and began practicing yoga in the early 1980s. The pain was still evident but became bearable, not nearly so intense. He continued with chiropractic care, although less and less frequently, and stepped up his practice of yoga. Today he is pain-free and maintains alignment through yoga.

Durán explains that movement is related to wellness on several levels. It enhances our ability to concentrate and focus. It also changes the chemistry in our bodies as we release toxins through perspiration, breathing and other eliminatory functions. Movement maintains and increases our range of motion, enabling our bodies to function well in a wide variety of activities. It helps fight the effects of gravity on our bodies and creates space between the bones, thus decompressing the spine and skeleton (which can get compressed each day by poor posture and a variety of other stressors). Just think about how difficult it is for a nerve to function when there is inadequate space between two vertebrae. Movement in this way ultimately supports the nervous system, relieving pressure on the nerves and allowing them to function without hindrance.

Another benefit of movement is the way it helps the body work through stress. In a stress response, our sympathetic (fight-or-flight) nervous system, part of the autonomic, or involuntary, nervous system (see Table 1 that follows), is engaged: We experience shortness of breath, a rush of adrenaline, an increased heart rate and higher blood pressure, and decreased circulation and production of "feel good" brain chemicals. We become disconnected from our bodies—which is important if we are, say, getting ready to fight or run from a wild animal. When the threat is averted, our bodies are supposed to return to a relaxed state. Unfortunately, in contemporary society, we tend to engage our stress response continually, to real or imagined threats (our bodies truly don't know the difference), and we tend to stay there, never returning to that relaxed state.

Constant anxiety, lack of rest and a poor diet all contribute to a prolonged stress response. By ingesting caffeine, highly processed foods, preservatives or artificial colors, flavors or sugar, we feed the fight-or-flight response. So many people today, in order to relax, self-medicate with alcohol or drugs like marijuana or prescription painkillers. These are attempts to engage the body's parasympathetic (rest-and-digest) nervous system response, which has the opposite physiological effect of fight or flight (see Table 1 that follows). The great news is that we don't need drugs or alcohol in order to relax—we can get the same results in safe, healthy ways.

**Table 1: Effect of autonomic nervous system response on body functions**

| Body Function | Autonomic Nervous System | |
|---|---|---|
| | Sympathetic (fight or flight) | Parasympathetic (rest and digest) |
| Breathing | ↑ | ↓ |
| Heart rate | ↑ | ↓ |
| Blood pressure | ↑ | ↓ |
| Circulation | ↓ | ↑ |
| "Feel good" brain chemicals— endorphins | ↓ | ↑ |
| Adrenaline | ↑ | ↔ |

**Table 2: Additional stress responses of the sympathetic nervous system**

| Body Function/Hormone | Increased | Decreased |
|---|---|---|
| Cortisol | X | |
| Heart rate | X | |
| Blood pressure | X | |
| Vasoconstriction | X | |
| Blood glucose levels | X | |
| Blood lipid levels | X | |
| Blood cholesterol levels | X | |
| LDL | X | |
| HDL | | X |
| Protein degradation of muscle and soft tissue | X | |
| Clotting factors | X | |
| Insulin resistance | X | |
| Fear, anxiety, depression | X | |
| Short-term memory | | X |
| Concentration (ADD/ADHD) | | X |
| Serotonin levels | | X |
| Noradrenaline levels (a neurotransmitter that boosts alertness and increases concentration) | X | |
| Sensory-system sensitivity, including pain | X | |
| Cellular immunity | | X |

| Body Function/Hormone | Increased | Decreased |
|---|---|---|
| Growth hormones | | X |
| Testosterone | | X |
| Luteinizing hormone (one of the hormones for reproductive functions; in women, triggers ovulation) | | X |
| Sex drive | | X |
| Digestion | | X |

## Get Moving, Get Stronger!

Movement is the best way to help our bodies work through the stress response with no harmful side effects. As we move our muscles, we burn sugar, increase respiration and increase circulation. The next time you're feeling stressed, take a long, hard walk and see whether you still feel as stressed afterward. But if you can't fit in a long walk, even two minutes of movement—jumping rope; doing jumping jacks, sit-ups or yoga poses; or dancing with abandon to music you love—can alter your body's stress state!

Adding regular aerobic exercise and strength training to your movement plan will support your overall health goals. With aerobic exercise, you don't have to rely on adrenaline because there's plenty of oxygen available to give you energy. According to the Mayo Clinic, aerobic exercise—even moderate exertion for 30 minutes a day—can have a positive impact on your health in a number of ways, including increased stamina, a stronger immune system, less anxiety and depression, and a lower risk of high blood pressure, diabetes, high cholesterol and heart disease.[1] I've already mentioned a few aerobic exercises, such as walking, jumping rope and dancing. These activities, along with running and swimming, are free or inexpensive ways to get moving.

Strength training can help you burn calories more efficiently by reducing body fat and increasing lean muscle mass (which diminishes with age).[2] It can also lower your risk of osteoporosis by increasing bone density; protect your joints and improve flexibility; and reduce symptoms of arthritis. You don't need to use much weight to have an impact; nor does strength training need to be costly. You can use your own body weight (such as with sit-ups and push-ups) or resistance bands for very effective strength building. Individual free weights are another inexpensive option.

In order to maximize your exercise results without over-stressing your body, it's important to monitor your heart rate—measured as beats per minute—to keep it within the target range. According to the American Heart Association, your target heart rate is 50 percent to 85 percent of your maximum heart rate, which is generally considered to be 220 minus your age.[3] Aim to keep your rate at the lower end of your target heart rate if you are less fit, and build up over time.

Once you know your target heart rate, how do you know whether you're in the range? You can wear a heart-rate monitor watch, but good ones aren't exactly a shoestring item. Instead you can manually take your pulse. Follow these instructions from the Cleveland Clinic[4]:

1. Place the tips of your index, second and third fingers on the palm side of your other wrist below the base of the

thumb. Or place the tips of your index and second fingers on your lower neck on either side of your windpipe.

2. Press lightly with your fingers until you feel the blood pulsing beneath your fingers. You may need to move your fingers around slightly up or down until you feel the pulsing.

3. Use a watch with a second hand, or look at a clock with a second hand.

4. Count the beats you feel for 10 seconds. Multiply this number by six to get your heart rate (pulse) per minute.

**A word of caution:** Before you begin a new exercise regimen, be sure to discuss your plans with your doctor.

## Lessons From Eastern Practices

Most people are breathing only at about 30 percent of their lung capacity, which dramatically reduces the oxygen they have available for basic bodily functions and for energy in general. Eastern systems of exercise, such as tai chi and yoga, and many of the martial arts are focused on the breath. The breath is literally the anchor to the movement. Deep, diaphragmatic breathing in certain ratios—in which the abdominal muscles move the organs out of the way slightly as you drop your diaphragm and fully expand your lungs, then compress the diaphragm as you fully exhale and the organs move back into place—can take you from a fight-or-flight nervous system response to a rest-and-digest response. It also massages the internal organs. In addition, it makes you present to right now, right here, to yourself.

It's impossible to move and not breathe, and as we know from Chapter 2, breathing deeply is a key wellness practice. When yoga instructors remind students to breathe, they are leading them to switch over to a parasympathetic nervous system response: Heart rate and blood pressure decrease, carbon dioxide and toxins are moved out of the body, the cells become fully oxygenated, and the chemical components of emotions are released in order to be flushed out of the body.

### Chiropractic Medicine: Movement and the Nervous System

"When one provides a human being with the natural ingredients it needs as a self-regulating, self-healing organism and removes the interferences to these innate abilities, the result is health and healing within the genetic limits of that human being."

—Dr. James L. Chestnut

"While other professions are concerned with changing the environment to suit the weakened body, chiropractic is concerned with strengthening the body to suit the environment."

—Dr. B. J. Palmer

A chiropractor is a board-qualified, licensed doctor whose training includes eight years of study, including an internship, prior to entering private practice.

Chiropractic care emphasizes the importance of the spine and nervous system to your overall health. Most people know that you can visit a chiropractor if you have back pain or headaches, but many do not realize that chiropractic care supports the body's ability to heal from a variety of other types of disease. Chiropractic care is conservative, seeking a drug-free, holistic approach to healing whenever possible. Its aim is to restore normal physiological function of the entire body by addressing nutrition, exercise and lifestyle choices and making adjustments to the spine that provide optimum spinal motion and support the nervous system's ability to function well. Chiropractic also has a spiritual connection through the laying on of hands, which directly integrates the powerful and natural healing energy fields that make up your body and the universe. Most important, chiropractic care is a partnership between the doctor and your body, mind and spirit, co-creating wellness.

Chiropractic is based, in part, on the belief that wellness depends on a healthy, well-functioning nervous system. The skull and the spinal vertebrae protect the most important and fragile organs of the nervous system: the brain and spinal cord. The spinal cord has 31 pairs of spinal nerves that exit the spinal column, or backbone, and affect every system in the body. The spine also provides weight-bearing support for the upright position. When the spine is aligned and healthy, the nervous system can operate optimally. When the spine is out of alignment, the ability of the nervous system to function properly is diminished and the stage is set for conditions of disease. When the body cannot communicate optimally within itself, it cannot function as well within its environment, nor can it respond as well to injury, illness or stress.

The nervous system consists of two principal parts: the central nervous system and the peripheral nervous system. The central nervous system is made up of the brain and spinal cord. The peripheral nervous system, which connects the brain and spinal cord with all the tissues of the body, consists of the somatic and autonomic systems. The autonomic nervous system—which has two components, the previously discussed sympathetic and parasympathetic responses (see Table 1)—carries out involuntary activities such as heartbeat, digestion and circulation. The somatic system (voluntary movement) includes the neurons connected with skeletal muscles, skin and sense organs. It consists of efferent nerves, also known as motor neurons, which are responsible for sending brain signals for muscle contraction.

Chiropractors believe that the body can and does maintain wellness and strong functioning provided it is not compromised. They understand the close communication among the nervous, immune and endocrine (hormone) systems, and they can use their expertise to help patients maintain a non-irritated nervous system by making sure the neck, spine and pelvis are functioning optimally. Chiropractors don't just treat the spine; they also address lifestyle issues such as nutrition and hydration, exercise, elimination of environmental toxins, and other practices that promote wellness—like the ones in this book.

Chiropractic care is very important in keeping the body moving well and in keeping messages moving through the nervous system. Accidents, falls, stress, tension, overexertion and illness may hinder the spine's ability to move with ease and cause subluxations, or minor displacements, of vertebrae to develop. These changes can irritate spinal nerves, which in turn can lead to malfunctions in various areas of the body, affecting the way the organs and organ systems operate and resulting in decreased immune system function and chronic disease. (See Table 3 that follows)

**Table 3: Possible effects of a spinal subluxation on different areas of the body**

| Section of the Spinal Cord | Areas of the Body Affected | Possible Effects or Symptoms of a Subluxation |
|---|---|---|
| Cervical (top) | Blood supply to the head, brainstem, ears, eyes, sinuses, sympathetic nervous system | Headaches, nervousness, dizziness, anxiety, migraines, insomnia, allergies, head colds, high blood pressure, deafness, earaches, eye problems, fevers |
| | Face, nose, lips, mouth | Skin and gland problems |
| | Neck glands, shoulders, arm, wrists, hands, fingers | Laryngitis, sore throat, stiff neck, bursitis, thyroid issues, asthma, cough, pain, numbness, tingling in lower arms and hands |
| Thoracic (upper) | Heart, lungs, breast | Heart conditions, bronchitis, pneumonia, asthma |
| | Gall bladder, liver, digestive organs | Issues with Gall bladder, liver, indigestion, heartburn, ulcers, blood sugar |

| Section of the Spinal Cord | Areas of the Body Affected | Possible Effects or Symptoms of a Subluxation |
|---|---|---|
| Thoracic (upper) | Spleen, adrenals | Lowered resistance, allergies, hives, blood sugar issues, varicose veins, fatigue, low blood pressure, skin problems, asthma |
| | Kidneys | Kidney problems, hardening of the arteries, chronic tiredness, skin conditions |
| Lumbar (lower) | Intestines | Gas pains, sterility, constipation, colitis, diarrhea |
| Sacrum (bottom) | Sex organs, uterus, bladder, knees, prostate glands, lower back | Bladder troubles, cramps, miscarriages, bed-wetting, impotency, knee pains, sciatica, difficult urination, backaches, poor circulation in legs, swollen, weak ankles and arches, cold feet, leg cramps, spinal curvatures, hemorrhoids |

Support your skeletal and muscular health further by checking out this list of not-so-great movements, followed by a list of good-for-you activities.

## Activities to Avoid or Limit:

1. Sleeping on your stomach.
2. Sitting on your billfold.
3. Always carrying a bag on one side.
4. Standing with your weight on one foot.
5. Reading, studying or watching TV in bed while using poor posture—such as slouching, not having back support, or holding a book above your head.
6. Doing one-sided sports (always exercise both hands).
7. Cradling the phone between your shoulder and ear.
8. Watching television for extended periods of time.
9. Doing repetitive activities with your arms in front of you or overhead.
10. Using poor posture while sitting or standing for prolonged periods of time.

## Healthy Activities:

1. Use correct sleep posture—supporting the neck and hips
2. Park as far away as possible from the entrance.
3. Take the stairs.
4. Add movement into your life: Get up and move at least once an hour (stretching, marching in place, jumping rope, walking), as well as incorporate an exercise regimen.
5. Use good posture while reading or studying.
6. Sit on good work chairs.

7. Get regular chiropractic checkups.

8. Sit on a fitness ball while using good posture.

9. Make daily living tasks more physical, like exercise.

10. Take up hobbies that require physical exertion.

11. Work out with a friend or friends.

12. Do yoga, Pilates or gymnastics.

13. Set up situations so that proper posture is required, such as positioning mirrors in your car or items on your desk so that you can use them only when sitting properly.

14. Dance!

## The Wellness Paradigm

The goal of chiropractic care is not merely the healing of disease but the maintenance of lifelong, total body wellness. Chiropractors work with you to move from disease or disability toward total health through the wellness paradigm. Where are you in your life today, and in which direction are you moving?

### Table 4: Wellness Paradigm

| Wellness Paradigm | | |
|---|---|---|
| Premature Death | ← Neutral point → | Wellness |
| Disability | (no | Awareness |
| Symptoms | discernible | Education |
| Signs | illness or | Growth |
| | wellness) | |

When you and your chiropractor create your plan for whole-body wellness, it can be overwhelming, because he or she is advising you on many different aspects of your health and may have a number of different suggestions for you to implement. Read over the list of suggestions every day for the next week, with no intention of implementing every single thing right away—simply to let your mind reinforce long-term goals. Do this for a week and then choose the one or two suggestions that are most important to you and that you feel most comfortable incorporating into your life at that point.

After four to six weeks, review the original list that you and your chiropractor created. You may be surprised to find that you were able to implement more suggestions than you initially intended because your mind found ways to incorporate wellness without your forcing the issue. Once you have successfully implemented your initial choices, return to the list and choose suggestions to work on next. Move at your own pace, and don't become stressed or obsessed. Unless you are facing a severe health crisis, incorporating lifestyle changes at a slow and steady rate is the best strategy for maintaining your new, healthy habits throughout your life.

## Personal Stories

One of my clients, Lee Harris, is a successful businessman who has incorporated meaningful movement into his daily life. He works out early every morning before breakfast. Lee started his lifestyle change with the help of a personal trainer who came to his house three times a week, and he worked out on his own two additional days each week. Beginning a lifestyle change with a trainer or partner is a good idea to help you create new, healthy habits. We do better when we have encouragement and accountability. This is especially important when we're practicing a lifestyle that is different from society's norm, because we're surrounded by so many practices that are the opposite of what we are creating!

At one point Lee stopped his morning routine, which had been working very well for him, and tried exercising later in the day. He quickly found that this change didn't work for him at all, and he went back to getting in his exercise early in the day. This is a good thing to remember: When you find what works for you, stick with it. When you get to a place where things aren't working, for whatever reason, go back to your basics, to what worked well for you at one point. Chances are it will work for you again.

It's also important to remember that we are all individuals. Some of us are morning people—we function best first thing in the morning. Others are truly night owls because nighttime is when their bodies and minds kick into high gear, and their energy skyrockets. Don't try to force your body to be something other than what it's naturally inclined to be. You know what kind of person you are, so plan your workouts or daily routines at the optimal times for you. Set yourself up to succeed!

Lee will tell you today that he has abundant energy—he's never tired during the day like many of his colleagues. His regular routine includes 30 minutes of a cardiovascular workout and 30 minutes of weight training Monday through Friday, then 30 minutes of a cardiovascular workout one weekend day and 30 minutes of weight training the other weekend day. He has a home-gym circuit where he utilizes free weights and a fitness ball, which is excellent for balance.

Lee has been working out for 20 years. He knows it's an integral part of who he is and why he's healthy. He says, "If I don't work out, I'll feel the lethargy. I won't have nearly as much energy. I'll be 55 in March, and I want to be toned and fit. It's important for weight and blood-sugar management." And it's equally important for his overall wellness and happiness.

On vacation Lee is active, but he's not rigid about working out. He resumes his workouts upon returning home and finds that his body remembers. He says, "Discipline is not something someone else imposes on me. I have no problem getting up in the morning and working out because it's a choice *I* have made. A huge part of my life is about discipline—my anchor is the way I live my life."

Gina Danner is another client who is utilizing movement, along with other lifestyle commitments, to live well. Gina, a successful CEO, came to me in extreme stress and pain, the kind of pain that literally made her scream. She had herniated three discs in her neck. She had tried steroid epidurals, physical therapy and heavy-duty painkillers. In order to sleep at night, she would literally "have Vicodin with a vodka chaser." Traditional Western medicine was not working for her, so she was self-medicating with painkillers and alcohol— a dangerous combination.

Gina was looking for a plan of action to manage her health. To her it felt as if traditional medicine was simply experimenting with her. The theory seemed to be "This didn't work, so let's see if *this* does." At the end of the day, though, nothing was working! I devised a comprehensive, four-month wellness plan for Gina that included chiropractic care and lifestyle changes. During that time, she was able to release one of the people from her life who had been causing her extreme stress, and her pain became manageable. As Gina was able to move more, to become physically "unstuck," she was able to break free from her inertia in other areas of her life. This was significant, but Gina wanted more than that—she wanted wellness.

For the next two years, Gina "sort of" committed to a healthier way of life. She was 80 pounds overweight, and she said she wanted to focus on weight loss (though her attitude was still "Can't you just adjust my spine into place and make everything fine?"). Gina got orthotics that supported her feet and helped her spine be in alignment, and this enabled her to begin an exercise program without pain. She began a detoxi-fication diet, and she also started to work with a fitness trainer. She lost 20 pounds. Then she gained it back. Gina was "playing at" improving her lifestyle, but she was not really committed.

Finally, Gina got real clarity. She realized that changing her lifestyle was "not about dying; it's about living a rich life and being able to do whatever I want to do whenever I want to do it." Extreme stress in a variety of areas of her life—career, per-sonal, physical—had finally pushed her to take control. Sometimes that's what it takes. Gina got serious. I helped her see that she was worth the investment of her time and energy to learn and implement a healthy lifestyle. She decided to take a one-week wellness vacation to Canyon Ranch health spa in Lenox, Massachusetts, a place where she could learn to eat differently (especially to eliminate her sugar habit), deal with stress effectively (including biofeedback) and take time to truly relax. She returned with the tools, confidence and commitment she needed to succeed.

You don't have to go to Canyon Ranch health spa—which is not for a shoestring budget—in order to reap these rewards, however. In addition to following the healthy tips presented in this book, look for low-cost classes covering similar subjects that are offered by community centers, wellness centers, hospitals and churches.

It can be quite the "aha" moment for people when they realize that striving for mind-body-spirit wellness is about prolonging and enhancing life rather than preventing or fighting disease. Gina had literally hurt every single day. She could not sleep. Her life felt out of her control. But when she took charge of her own health, things really changed. Now Gina has no daily pain, only residual pain now and then from her neck. In addition to other healthy lifestyle commitments, she burns 500 calories each day through exercise, spending 45 minutes doing a combination of cardio work on the Stairmaster and interval training on the elliptical.

Gina says, "There are only a few things in your life that you truly can control, and these include what you do with your body and what you put in your mouth. When you live as if you are a healthful, intent, fit person, eventually you will become a healthful, intent, fit person. It's not about the weight—it's about fully living my life."

Karen Zecy, another friend and client, is a longtime supporter of Women's Intersport Network for Kansas City (WIN for KC), an organization that promotes women's lifelong participation in sports and fitness. At the WIN for KC banquet in

2009, Karen's friends had suggested that she participate in the upcoming triathlon that WIN for KC sponsors each year. She resisted, proclaiming that she couldn't; after all, she hadn't done any of that—running, swimming, biking—in years! Karen was 52 and in shape but did not exercise consistently. But eventually she was convinced to sign up; after all, she figured, she had four months to train. She decided that the triathlon would be a good incentive to start exercising more frequently. And besides, she had told everyone she'd do it, so she had to follow through.

The first day she took out her bike, she couldn't even get up a little hill in her neighborhood. She had to stop, get off the bike and walk it up the hill. The next day she made it a little farther. By the end of the week she could make it up the hill. When Karen first started running, she also couldn't get very far without having to stop and walk for a while. She found the swimming leg of the workout easier.

Karen needed all the positive encouragement she could get. She loaded up her iPod with energetic, fast-paced music, lectures from motivational speakers and audio books about strong, amazing women. She found it exhilarating to have the quiet time alone while being inspired. She also called friends who would bike or run with her. Her support network of friends and family, combined with the energy and motivation of the music and stories she listened to while training, pushed her through the lull that most of us experience when we first make this kind of shift in our lives.

Early on, there had been a preparatory orientation of WIN for KC triathlon participants at YWC. The athletes were given tips on what and when to eat, the importance of keeping hydrated, and how and when to stretch. Karen applied all that she learned but still started to feel pain in one of her legs. She visited me for an adjustment, and over time she began to learn the differences in pain—when she had just pushed herself physically versus when there was truly something wrong. She also realized that it was important to have regular chiropractic care and monitor the impact of the workouts on her body.

Karen was also experiencing fantastic positive changes in her body. She was sleeping better, was well hydrated, had increased stamina and felt the stress melt away. She felt physically and mentally energized. She only lost about 10 pounds but felt a tremendous increase in strength throughout her body. She also became more conscious of what she was eating. The emotional impact was important too. Karen found a new level of confidence as she achieved a victory over negative self-talk.

WIN for KC opened a practice course, and Karen came in last, but she did not let that stop her. Instead, she increased her training. When the next opportunity to practice part of the course—bike and run—came around, she did it and this time was not last. On triathlon day, Karen finished in the middle of the pack! She was so proud she had finished, she wanted to tattoo her body marking (the participant's number, written with marker) all the way down her arm. Fortunately, though, reason prevailed! She participated in her second triathlon just a month later.

Karen, who has a new goal of staying triathlon-ready, continues her workouts. Physical activity gives her the energy, stamina, flexibility and sense of "feel good" that she wants in her everyday life. She actually enjoys the cleansing power of sweat. She has also noticed how her new level of fitness allows her to do more in her everyday life. It also makes doing other types of exercise, like yoga, easier. Her lower back pain is gone, as are her occasional headaches. Biking has become her passion! Her husband and friends frequently join her for bike rides. Karen is grateful for her health—and her ability to *move*—more than ever. She celebrates being healthy every day.

Fred Pryor is a dear friend and successful businessman, and one of my personal inspirations. He is 75 and fit, has no health issues and takes no medications. How did he do it?

Like most of us, Fred was an active child and young adult. He was busy playing out what was in his imagination and later channeled that energy into sport, track and weights. As he moved into adulthood, he became preoccupied with graduate school, a wife and a child. He stopped exercising and his body changed.

Fred's career required a tremendous amount of energy. He traveled all over the United States and presented 225 all-day seminars during any given year. He would be up early, setting up the training room, on his feet training and presenting all day, then would pack it all up and jump on a plane to the next city to do it all again. On the weekends he was home to be a husband and father. There was no downtime.

Fred wanted to regain the health, fitness and energy of his boyhood. He was motivated by his desire for something positive, not out of what he "ought to" or "should" do. As Fred has said, "Motivation is the anticipation of achievement." He began running again. He got up early each morning in whatever city he was in and ran 45 minutes. It relieved the tension, helped him cope with the stress, and built his stamina to help him make it through the long days and weeks of his job.

Remember that Fred was doing this in the late 1950s and early 1960s. There wasn't the fitness culture we have today, with specially designed running shoes and matching workout outfits. Fred wore tennis shoes, swim trunks and a T-shirt to go running, and he always got a few looks while riding the hotel elevator. As he ran through strange neighborhoods around the country in the wee hours of the morning, it was not uncommon for a police car to follow him awhile or pull up alongside to see what he was up to. Fred didn't let the strange, judgmental looks from others keep him from what he wanted to do for his health.

The years Fred was doing this were also the dawn of the fast-food era in American culture. Fred soon realized that eating a diet of fast food, particularly on the road, was not helping move him toward his goal of being healthier and fit. He began rigorously watching what he ate. Initially he just cut out the fast food. Over the years he became a strict vegetarian, and he continues eating that way to this day. He also became acutely aware of his dependence on caffeine and how it was keeping him from being able to truly rest and re-energize. One day, stepping off the plane, he realized that he was so exhausted, he could hardly move his feet. At the same time, he was so wired from the caffeine that he could hardly close his eyes. He quit cold turkey and hasn't looked back.

Over time, Fred developed habits and patterns that supported his health goals. Now, at 75, he often hears friends say,

"If I knew I would live this long, I would have taken better care of myself!" Fred didn't know that he would live this long, but he has, and he wants to be able to continue living the life he's always wanted. He still wants options in his life. Fred is fond of saying, "Only the disciplined are free." Only when you have the discipline and the mindfulness to take care of your body—the vehicle of your mind and spirit—are you truly free to pursue your passions.

Fred's exercise routine has evolved over time. His current daily routine includes 15 minutes of breathing exercises and meditation; a run, walk or hike; weight lifting three times a week; and a sauna (infrared or steam) and swimming a few times a week. There are a few other activities he throws in for variety, including yoga class twice a week. He feels that yoga is very important to keeping his body flexible, strong and open for the energy to flow.

Fred encourages us not to focus on how accomplished we are in our fitness journey, but just to ask if we're on the right path. He calls his approach to life "optioneering," or engineering his options. Throughout his life, health and fitness have provided him with options, energy and well-being to do just about anything he has desired. Fred says, "We think we make our decisions, when in reality our decisions make us." He made the decision to live well as long as he is on this earth, and he still focuses on that boyhood energy and vitality as inspiration. Daily exercise and movement have been critical to his success and mind-body-spirit wellness.

## Practical Tips for Your Journey

Gina Danner has several strategies pertaining to movement and beyond that have helped her take control of her wellness lifestyle:

1. Above all, be honest with yourself about where you are at this moment in time. Tell your chiropractic doctor your real-diet day, not your best-diet day. Be honest with yourself. Get on the scale every single day; don't let the liquid pounds become solid pounds.

2. Move! Move! Move! Make exercise a priority in your life, wherever it fits into your schedule: before breakfast, during lunchtime, right before you pick the kids up from school or after you put them to bed. To keep track of how much you are moving, consider wearing a pedometer. You can find them for under $25.

3. Switch from coffee or soda pop to green tea.

4. Surround yourself with people who have similar values. The biggest thing is to keep your life peaceful. Try to be cautious about those people you let into your life. Release those who suck energy, or else change the way you are with them in that relationship; for example, invite them to be with you in a new, healthy activity.

5. Remember that it's all about changing habits. Reject old, unhealthy patterns and create new patterns. Start with a small goal, such as "From one holiday until the next holiday, I'll exercise 15 minutes each day," for example, until the exercise becomes a habit. Structure is a good thing; it allows you to let go.

People do best when they have certain boundaries around them. Wouldn't you rather be in control of your boundaries? You have a choice now; you might not have a choice someday in the future. The choice might be made for you—by your body, say, when it can no longer do what you want or need it to do. Do you want to be the crumpled-up 80-year-old, or do you want to be the one who is still playing tennis and swimming?

6. Pay deep attention to your breathing. When you are under stress, try taking 10 deep, diaphragmatic breaths.

7. Practice gratitude! Realize that we have a greater impact than we realize. (Gina lives her gratitude by giving back to others, by charity work and by sharing from her abundance.)

## Your Space

Use this page to make notes and write your own reflections on moving your body.

# Chapter 4

# Free Your Space

Clutter handcuffs you to the past. It sets obstacle after obstacle in the way of your goals, saps your energy, and prevents you from seeing clearly and moving forward. Clutter comes in many forms: overflowing physical stuff; people or objects that hold bad memories or energy; fears, doubts and regrets; and toxins in the body. The good news is you can clean house, literally and figuratively, and be free! Do you wonder whether your mind-body-spirit is cluttered? Ponder the questions below and read on.

## Questions to Consider

∞ Do you find that you're in the same place you were 10 years ago, sharing the same stories, voicing the same complaints?

∞ Can you remember the last day you spent all by yourself? How did you feel? Peaceful? Anxious? Did you find yourself searching for things to distract you?

∞ Do you have trouble sleeping? Is your bedroom clean and organized?

∞ Do you have so many clothes that when you purchase a new item, you struggle to find space in your closet?

∞ Where in your life are you creating white space? Consider your calendar, your physical space, your mind, your relationships and your connection to Spirit.

∞ Do you experience frequent diarrhea or constipation, or alternate between the two?

෨ How do you feel when the phone rings and someone needs your attention?

෨ Are there any relationships in your life that are no longer good for you, that you may need to release?

෨ Do you lack focus? Does your mind seem scattered? Do you struggle with "mind chatter?" Are you able to name it and let it go?

෨ Is the way you care for your insides reflected in your outside environment? How?

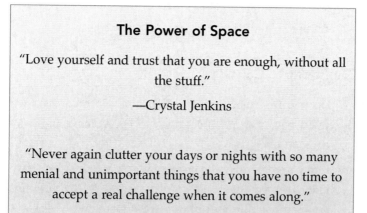

### The Power of Space

"Love yourself and trust that you are enough, without all the stuff."

—Crystal Jenkins

"Never again clutter your days or nights with so many menial and unimportant things that you have no time to accept a real challenge when it comes along."

—Og Mandino

You may experience many different types of clutter during your life: There is spiritual clutter, which can keep you from being who you truly are. You may have mental or emotional clutter stemming from the beliefs of your parents which leaves you stuck in the past or worried about the future and unable to fully enjoy the present. You may also have clutter in your body, such as toxins stored in your liver or fat cells, or simply foods in your diet that don't work with your body chemistry. Any of these elements can make it harder for your body to function.

One of the most powerful things you can do to support your own wellness is the regular elimination of what does not support or nurture you. Perhaps your bed is unmade, and all the surfaces of your bedroom are piled with laundry and paperwork. This creates an unsettled, unclear vibration in the room that makes it difficult to sleep well. Maybe your desk is cluttered, affecting your ability to think clearly and creatively. Or perhaps your car is dirty and in need of minor repair, like windshield wipers that need to be replaced. This creates a low level of ongoing anxiety that affects your day-to-day ability to function well. Similarly, a cluttered closet jammed full of clothes that you hope to fit into someday keeps you from loving who and where you are right now.

And then there is the clutter of things that people put between themselves and other people, and between themselves and new experiences. Do you touch your partner lovingly as you sleep, or do you always have a pet or pillow between you? Is there so much going on in your calendar that you have no white space, no downtime and no space for something new to come into your life?

Clutter disconnects you from yourself, from your heart, and keeps you living a life in which you are not paying attention. You live looking in at all the mess, and you never have the energy to look out and around you, able to access what could bring you a better life. Clutter feeds a mindless way of living that keeps you mired in chaos and can lead to many forms of disease. But don't despair: Wellness increases naturally and easily as you get rid of the clutter. And cleaning out your life doesn't have to happen all at once, in one huge cleansing session; it can and does happen bit by bit.

Also, know that when you de-clutter your environment and your emotional self, you get rid of the noise that can keep you from being able to hear your inner wisdom or connect to a higher self or God. De-cluttering other parts of your life gives your mind and body, literally and figuratively, the space to be open, to have a dialogue with God, to connect with your spirit and receive the gifts of the Spirit.

## Free Your Space the Feng Shui Way

Feng shui is a Chinese system of placement and arrangement of buildings, rooms, objects, etc., according to the flow of energy in the environment, so as to increase well-being. Feng shui teaches that your outside world is a reflection of what's going on inside. You arrange your space and your things to support who you are and who you are becoming. When you create order out of chaos, bringing structure to your life and taking care of all the so-called mundane needs each day, you free up space for creative thinking and problem solving.

Transformational life coach Marlene Sohl, who is also a feng shui consultant, suggests that you begin to look at your surroundings by asking yourself, "When I come into this space, does my energy rise, is it neutral or does it go down?" You can also do this exercise with specific objects, by picking up each one and asking, "When I interact with this object, does my energy rise, is it neutral or does it go down?" You can even do this with a gift. Just because someone gives you a present does not mean that you have to keep it. Decide whether it brings you good energy; if not, regift it. Your "trash" may be someone else's treasured item—and as long as you refuse to release it, they cannot enjoy it!

It is said that nature abhors a vacuum. So as you make space and then stand in faith and trust, certain that something positive will come into your life to replace what you have released, you invite new opportunities, new people and new experiences into your world. You open yourself up to seeing and moving into the next facet of your life, and you are able to move along your path gently.

Let's consider your home. As Sohl points out, the most important thing is to create an environment that supports you. Everything has a vibration. Wood used to be a tree; bricks used to be earth. Because everything is energy, your home is a living thing! Everything in your house has a specific energy. When you treat your home with respect, you also treat yourself with respect. You had a certain energy about you when you acquired each item in your home, and you continue to feel that energy later.

The easiest way to clear out clutter is to take everything out of the room (or pantry, closet, drawer, shelf or other space) that you can. Put back only what you use or feel you need, or that has a good kind of sentiment that you want to hold on to. Get rid of the rest.

You can do this with clothing too. (We use only a small fraction of our clothes anyway.) Take out all the clothes from your closet. Try on each item and look in the mirror. Ask, "Is this me now?" Realize that when you put on an article of clothing, you are taken back to a particular time and place in your life. It may or may not represent who you are today. Put back only those clothes that you wear!

You probably already know that this process is also helpful when you want to change the way you eat. You cannot
support a change in your diet as long as your fridge and
pantry are full of junk, so one of the first things you do is clear
your space of the clutter (unhealthy foods).

Don't become overwhelmed! Make small changes; remind
yourself that things did not get this way overnight. You did
not gain weight all at once; you gained it one doughnut at a
time. When you're moving toward a healthier way of eating,
making one small change a day makes a big difference over
time. Likewise, eliminating clutter a little bit each day will
ultimately lead to huge results.

Many of us have a tendency to give away our energy to
others. This is admirable but can become dangerous if we get
depleted. We cannot take care of anybody else if we don't first
look after ourselves! Eliminating clutter in its various forms
provides us with energy and focus, bringing wellness, balance and the ability to provide sustained care for the people
and situations in our lives.

## Consider a Detox

Clearing out other areas of your life automatically benefits
the body because you have created more space for yourself,
resulting in deeper, easier breathing. You also move more easily because you are no longer symbolically carrying the
weight of objects and feelings that you have shed. Feeling
lighter and unburdened, in turn, can motivate you to take
better care of yourself by exercising, eating better and following the other wellness practices detailed in this book.

To assist your body even further, think about removing toxins through a detox program. There are several ways to cleanse the body, and you can find a number of detox products at wellness centers and health food stores. Detoxifying cleanses, however, are not for everyone. The process, which can be costly, takes a lot of discipline, so before you perform one, it is very important to be ready emotionally and to know why you are doing it.

You can detox anytime, but I recommend doing it during a change of seasons. How long you conduct the detox cleanse (anywhere from three to 21 days) is also a personal choice. The holistic health and nutrition coach at YWC likes to do a 10-day cleanse, and many of our clients find this length of time very doable. If you want to try a short, simple detox, check out this three-day detox that we often recommend at YWC:

Days 1 and 3: Eat only vegetables and fruit (raw or cooked).

Day 2, liquid fast: Consume only vegetable juices, mineral broth and herbal teas. If you can't tolerate a liquid fast, add in a few vegetables and fruit.

**A few suggestions for a successful detox:**

🔸 Before you start a cleanse, eat very simple, whole, organic foods (or "clean eating") to help reduce some of the symptoms that the detox may cause, such as headaches, fatigue, feeling more emotional and foggy thinking.

🔸 Be prepared! Do your grocery shopping and prepare veggies, soups or salads ahead of time.

~

§ Do not chew gum. The digestive process starts when chewing prompts the body to secrete enzymes into the gastrointestinal tract.

§ If you experience symptoms of hypoglycemia, or low blood sugar—such as anxiety, sweating, dizziness or confusion—during Day 2, consider taking five tablets of Spirulina three times a day. It's available at wellness and health food stores.

§ Get adequate sleep during the detox.

§ Drink copious amounts of water, a minimum of 80 ounces per day.

§ On Day 2, do not take your regular daily supplements.

§ If you must break the fast on Day 2, eat watermelon by itself or combine it with apples (leave the skin on) in a smoothie or blended soup.

§ Engage in any of these activities to help draw out toxins further through sweating or deep breathing: yoga, walking or other light exercise; breathing exercises or meditation (see Chapter 2); soaking in an Epsom salt bath; or sitting in an infrared sauna, if you have access to one.

**A word about colonics:** Another option for detoxing the body, particularly the digestive system, is getting a colonic, or colon hydrotherapy. Colonics will quickly clean out the colon, and I do recommend them to certain patients. They are not inexpensive, however (an average session can cost $85), and there are better, long-term ways to create a cleaner, lighter state of being.

~

## Clear Your Mind

Licensed professional counselor Crystal Jenkins explains that an emotionally cluttered mind is commonly filled with "woulda, coulda, shoulda" thoughts of fear, doubt and worry. There is the questioning of decisions you could or should make and the fear of making the wrong one. The emotionally cluttered mind is desperate to control the uncontrollable—the dance between the past and future—and the ego tricks you into thinking you have that control. All of which distracts you from being present!

Take a real look at where that mental chatter comes from. For many of us, it's the same voices we heard in childhood—either from Mom and Dad or our brothers and sisters. We carry those thoughts into adulthood and continue the same behavior and beliefs. We do what our parents taught us to do in order to connect to them in childhood. Our parents' attitudes and beliefs constitute the voices that make up our mental "committee."

Awareness is key, Jenkins explains. When you experience mental clutter, identify where and from whom you learned to live in the past or the future. Separate that learned clutter from you! Come back to what is true at this moment. Connect in the present to your body, breath and feelings—your truth in this moment. For the sake of your well-being, you need to be present to what *is*, to your own knowing. For many of us, however, the fear is that if we stop doing and are simply still, we might have to come face-to-face with what we feel, which can be scary because we will have to give up control.

Feelings are messy and uncomfortable. Most of us weren't taught in childhood to embrace and accept our emotional capacity. In fact, we were taught to shut it down or learned to express the extremes of emotions such as anger, leading to hurt and pain. Feelings in adults are not accepted as productive and therefore are not validated as important, so we suppress them and deny that they even exist. We skim the water of life, obeying the chatter in our heads in an attempt to quiet the committee. But in fact, we just continue to give the committee power, feeding the monster!

You were born whole, absolutely complete. As your personality was formed, you developed that committee, along with the belief that you needed it to guide you on the right path. The key is remembering that the present, the right now, is where you are truly connected to your wisdom, your wholeness. It is all you have control over. Ask yourself in the moment, "What do I feel? Where in my body do I feel it?" Place your hand on that place and connect to you. The body is always in the present moment.

Stop skimming the water of life. There are buried treasures below the surface. Embrace every moment. You will remember more about what you did and how it felt. You will experience a deeper connection to life, those you love and yourself.

## Emotional Development in Children

No matter what you do, developing their emotional selves is something your children will have to navigate. Do the best you can, allowing them to be authentically who they are. Set good boundaries, then allow them as much freedom and expression as possible. The emotional self is the place that gets arrested in development. The intellect gets fed all day, every day, but children need extra support for the development of their emotional selves.

Realize that even with the best parents, at some point children are going to perceive a "disconnect" with their parents. This is about our children's growth, and it's not our place to get involved in that journey beyond creating a safe place with set boundaries. Oftentimes, as parents, we try to re-create our own story through our children's lives, to make it better, but this process really is—and needs to be—all about them!

Remind yourself that the greatest love songs, poems, stories and art all come out of struggle. It's about personal transformation. Do the best you can, then step out of your kids' stuff. Let them have their own journeys. You can offer solid support, provide good instructions, and model nice, clear boundaries. Then let them do it. It's hard—in fact, it's one of the hardest things about being a parent. But it's the right thing to do.

## Personal Stories

Lea McGuire is a witty, intelligent, stylish, competent woman in her late 40s. She has a great laugh, deep intuition and powerful energy. Today Lea is great fun to be around. But she wasn't always so free. When she first came to see me for chiropractic care for back pain, she insisted that no one at my practice hug her because in her world, that was always and only an invitation to sex.

Lea experienced various forms of abuse during her childhood. In addition, her mother was always suffering from one illness or another, a pattern that her brother emulated. There were numerous illnesses and injuries, as well as other drama. Lea had a dysfunctional relationship with her father, an angry man whom she either avoided or tried to distract with humor.

Lea's early religious training brought her only shame and guilt. She was taught that she should respect her parents no matter what, and that it was a sin to ever have bad thoughts about them. She lived in a state of constant vigilance, never feeling safe, always trying to make sense out of craziness, and feeling guilty about any anger.

As an adult, Lea became a very successful workaholic, driven by fear: fear of failure, fear of being hurt again. She pushed her emotions down deep, and she ran away from relationships. She developed multiple sclerosis. Lea never allowed herself any quiet, keeping the TV on at all times and infusing her life with noise so that she wouldn't have to deal with the thoughts that would surface in times of silence. She couldn't stand to be alone, and she couldn't allow herself to get close to others. Lea continued to struggle with her parents' actions. She also struggled with blame and pain, and not understanding and not forgiving.

Lea was stuck because of mental and emotional clutter. Her constant devotion to her work had also become a kind of clutter, keeping her from processing what she needed to in order to become well. Lea was given time to deal with her clutter, in the form of a layoff from work and four lost jobs in a row (funny how that happens in life sometimes). I suggested that she attend the Hoffman Process—an experiential course in forgiveness and spirituality that provides a framework for understanding human behavior and development—in order to release her clutter. While the process is not inexpensive, scholarships are available. You can also read about how to overcome the negative behavior patterns that are sometimes passed down from generation to generation in the booklet *A Path to Personal Freedom and Love,* available by free download at the Hoffman Web site (see Additional Wellness Resources in the back pages of this book). And keep in mind that seeing a counselor can be very beneficial and is frequently covered by health insurance.

Lea did attend the course, and she began to understand her parents a bit more. She realized that she was adopting many of her parents' patterns of behavior and treating herself the same way. Through all the work she did with Hoffman and counseling, she undertook the process of forgiving them and herself. She did additional work with a spiritual teacher and began dreaming new dreams to fill the space left vacant as she removed her mental and emotional clutter. In the space created after she lost her jobs, Lea decided to start her own business, specializing in organizational design and development. She now helps businesses de-clutter, streamline, train and focus. The space she freed up in her personal life is being filled with a new relationship of love. Lea says, "He is the first person I've ever really loved. I can actually say to him 'I love you' and mean it. What's going to happen, I have no clue. But I'm not scared now. I'm sleeping fine. I'm not worrying about what's going to happen to me." And nowadays, Lea is completely comfortable with hugs; in fact, she shares them regularly.

Another one of my clients, transformational life coach Marlene Sohl, whose thoughts on feng shui appear earlier in the chapter, became interested in exploring colonics, something I frequently recommend. It made sense to her that toxins could get stuck in our bodies and affect the tissue in which they are stored. After she had a colonic, she started noticing the unpleasant reactions she was having to certain foods. She began to listen to her body more and more. Marlene says, "When I ate wheat, I would get stupid! My brain would simply *not* work right; I would get foggy. The same thing was happening with milk, yogurt—all dairy. I realized I was eating something not good for my body chemistry, and by doing that I was clogging up my internal system. This forced my body to work harder, using energy that I could have used for something else. Once I eliminated dairy and wheat from my diet, I had a lot more energy, I thought more clearly and I simply felt better."

Marlene also had a powerful experience as she made some changes in her home life. A few years after her divorce, she realized that her apartment just did not feel like a reflection of her. It felt like a place that someone was ready to leave at any moment. That represented the way she had lived her life during her unhappy marriage, but it wasn't how she was living now. She decided to hire a feng shui consultant, and this expert helped Marlene make some simple changes, moving some of her artwork around and organizing her space in a way that worked for her. Suddenly things began to feel more settled. People who visited would say, "Wow, I could live here!" Marlene eliminated a few items and moved others, and now, instead of a temporary place of lodging, Marlene has a home.

Gina Danner, whom we first met in Chapter 3, is another client who had to eliminate a kind of clutter to make her life work better. The herniated discs in her neck were causing her such pain that she could not sleep without painkillers and alcohol, and during the day the pain literally made her scream. She came to see me after not getting relief from the traditional medical community. As part of her treatment, I encouraged her to review her home and work life and remove those things, people and experiences that were depleting her energy and causing clutter, physically and emotionally.

Gina fired an employee who was causing her and others in the company extreme stress. One week later her pain was significantly reduced, and she was on the path to feeling well again. She eliminated sugar from her diet. She learned a healthier way of eating, replacing soda pop with green tea and water. She also got rid of physical clutter in her life. And the changes were phenomenal—not only dramatically reduced pain, but also weight loss, increased energy and focus, and a new ability to live her life the way she wanted.

## Practical Tips for Your Journey

1. Identify your mental and emotional clutter. Ask yourself, "What occupies my thoughts, my attention? What past hurts, needs and emotions from childhood am I still carrying around as an adult?"

2. Realize the ways in which this clutter is really the "committee" of Mom and Dad showing up in your life today.

3. Ask yourself, "How does this clutter serve me, and how it does not serve me?"

4. Start moving out ways of thinking that no longer serve you. Replace old ways with new ones that support who

you are and who you are becoming. As you do so, start moving out physical items that no longer serve you. Notice how the two are often connected.

5. Ask yourself, "Who am I without my clutter?" Remind yourself that clutter reveals a lack of belief that your needs will be met. Begin to design or redesign your life your way. Take your time, and enjoy the process.

## Your Space

Use this page to make notes and write your own reflections on freeing your space.

_____

_____

_____

_____

_____

_____

_____

_____

_____

_____

_____

_____

_____

_____

# Chapter 5

# Go for the Greens

If I could recommend only one food group for you to incorporate into your diet for whole-body wellness, it would be vegetables, but especially greens. It is certainly crucial to include a wide variety of vegetables of all colors in your diet to make the most of the nutrients they provide. I will be focusing in this chapter on greens, however, because they have such tremendous health benefits and are all too often overlooked. Consider the following questions and then learn the top reasons to incorporate more greens into your diet. You will be surprised at the impact!

## Questions to Consider

∾ How many servings of vegetables do you eat each day, especially raw veggies? How many leafy green vegetables?

∾ How often do you experience congestion, viral infections or bacterial infections?

∾ Is your cholesterol high?

∾ Are your nails weak?

∾ How many times do you chew your food before swallowing? Do you eat mindfully?

∾ How often do you experience gas?

∾ Do you struggle with offensive breath or excessive belching, burping or bloating?

∾ Do you experience indigestion and fullness that lasts during eating and/or up to four hours after eating?

∾ Do you have difficulty losing weight?

∾ When you eat fiber, do you experience constipation?

∾ Do you experience easy bowel movements each day?

∾ Do you have diarrhea? Constipation? Alternating bouts of each?

∾ Do you use laxatives frequently?

∾ Are your stools hard, dry or small? Are they undigested, foul smelling, mucus-like, greasy or poorly formed?

∾ Does your tongue feel coated? Does it ever feel "fuzzy"?

∾ Do you find yourself urinating frequently, experiencing increased thirst or appetite?

## The Power of Greens

"Nothing will benefit human health and increase the chances for survival of life on Earth as much as the evolution to a vegetarian diet."
—Albert Einstein

"Greens are the primary food group that match all human nutritional needs most completely."
—Victoria Boutenko

Consider the color green. What comes to mind? I think of spring and summer, renewal, growth, abundance, vibrant life! Green plants provide oxygen, without which there would be no life as we know it. In Asian medicine, green is associated with creativity, emotional stability and the liver (which, among other things, supports wellness by filtering toxins from the blood).

Dark green leafy vegetables are veritable powerhouses of nutrition. They grow naturally from the earth, providing phytochemicals, vitamins and minerals that feed us on a cellular level. They are high in calcium, magnesium, iron, potassium, phosphorous, zinc and vitamins A, C, E and K. They are also filled with fiber and folic acid. According to the Institute for Integrative Nutrition, you can reap the following benefits by regularly eating dark leafy greens[1]:

- A stronger immune system
- Improved liver, gall bladder and kidney function
- Blood-sugar balance
- Blood purification
- Improved circulation
- Healthier intestinal flora
- A lower risk of cancer
- Greater energy
- A better mood, less susceptibility to depression
- Less congestion because of reduced mucus

Greens give cells what they need chemically so that they can function optimally. When we are healthy on a cellular level, we can sustain wellness in our organs and organ systems and as whole organisms. Cellular health begins with what we eat and drink and how able our bowels are to process what we put in our bodies.

## Time for a Gut Check!

Immune system function is largely bowel-related. A healthy gut absorbs nutrients, breeds healthy bacteria and communicates well with the nervous system, keeping the right balance of chemicals in the body for the health of neurotransmitters. The nervous system is the regulating entity that produces the immune response. Think of the small and large intestines as a long, flexible pipe winding through the abdominal cavity. This pipe cannot absorb nutrients when it is not healthy. It can even get clogged up like a bathroom pipe or kinked like a hose because of sunken posture, stress or what we eat. Wellness author Louise Hay has written about how even negative thoughts can clog up our pipes.

The bowels follow directions from the nervous system. As I discussed in Chapter 3, the nervous system controls and coordinates all bodily functions, including digestive processes. Research indicates that the nervous system is affected by chemistry and thought. Our bodies' chemical composition comes from the vitamins, minerals and other micronutrients we eat. If the intestines don't get enough nutrients, signals can't get back to the nervous system. With more than half the body's nerve cells in the gut, it would seem to be our second brain—or is it our first?

If the intestines are unhealthy, inflammation most likely exists somewhere in the body. It's important to reduce inflammation because it's the primary cause of the chronic diseases devastating our society, such as diabetes, cancer and heart disease. According to a study published in the November 2005 issue of *Alternative Therapies in Health and Medicine*, "Inflammation is now recognized as an overwhelming burden to the health care status of our population and the underlying basis of a significant number of diseases. The elderly generally bear the burden of morbidity and mortality, which may be reflective of elevated markers of inflammation resulting from decades of lifestyle choices. Lower cancer rates are associated with diets high in fiber, fruits, vegetables and tea."[2]

A diet rich in greens and other healthy foods can provide most of the nutrients. Your intestines, however, have to be able to absorb them. This information from the Institute for Integrative Nutrition explains how eating greens helps keep the gut healthy:

1. Greens are rich in digestive and antioxidant enzymes, which makes them perfectly digestible. Many of the foods we commonly eat never get fully digested; instead they sit in the bowels to rot, become toxic and block nutrient absorption. The enzymes in greens naturally help toxins release from the gut for elimination. When the intestines are cleaned out, they are able to do their job properly and absorb nutrients.

2. Greens help normalize the gut's elimination process. They contain potassium and cell salts. Potassium causes the bowels to contract, while salts cause them to expand. This contract-expand movement is what squeezes waste through the intestines for elimination, a process we all want to have work daily and easily.

3. Greens alkalize the body. Because of the typical American diet, we tend to have a more acidic digestive system. An overly acidic body is linked to the development of illness and disease, including cancer. Eating green leafy

vegetables balances the acidity and alkaline levels in the body. The blood needs a pH level of 7.4—higher than 7 is alkaline, and lower is acidic. Do you get indigestion? Your acidic levels are high.

The common response to indigestion is to take an antacid. Unfortunately, that neutralizes the acid and does not balance it, so your food is not properly digested—plus you're still acidic. Now you have the problem of undigested food clogging your gut and nutrients not being absorbed properly. Keeping your body pH-balanced by eating lots of greens will solve these problems. Added bonus: Greens alkalizing the gut also help regulate the passage of glucose, thus regulating blood sugar!

## A Wealth of Nutrients

YWC wellness advocate Shelly Murray, a graduate of the Institute for Integrative Nutrition and a certified holistic heath practitioner, explains, "Greens are the most nutrient-dense food we know. There is more protein in 100 calories of kale than in 100 calories of steak, and the protein in spinach is perfectly designed for ease of digestion." Dark green leafy vegetables are also the best and safest source of trace minerals, which barely exist in the processed foods we commonly eat. Trace minerals help build white blood cells called T-lymphocytes, or T-cells, which are critical to the body's ability to respond to disease. The body will use or release all the minerals it gets from vegetables, but it will often store unused minerals consumed via supplements, which can lead to a toxic buildup.

The following chart—based on information from SpectraCell Laboratories, a leader in micronutrient testing and testing for nutritional deficiencies—provides a list of key nutrients, ways that they affect the body, and good vegetable sources (especially greens):

**Table 5: Key nutrients and their properties (*Used with permission from SpectraCell Laboratories*)**

| Nutrient | What It Does/Body Systems It Benefits | Green and Other Vegetable Sources | Symptoms and Problems of Deficiency |
|---|---|---|---|
| VITAMIN E | Antioxidant; regulates oxidation reactions, stabilizes cell membrane, boosts immune function; protects against cardiovascular disease, cataracts and macular degeneration | Dark leafy greens, sweet potatoes, avocados, asparagus | Issues with skin or hair, rupturing of red blood cells, anemia, bruising, PMS, hot flashes, eczema, psoriasis, cataracts, wound healing, muscle weakness, sterility |
| CALCIUM | Strengthens bones and teeth; helps heart, nerves, muscles, body systems work properly; needs other nutrients to function | Broccoli, cabbage, dark leafy greens | Osteoporosis, osteomalacia, osteoarthritis, muscle cramps, irritability, acute anxiety, colon cancer risk |

| Nutrient | What It Does/ Body Systems It Benefits | Green and Other Vegetable Sources | Symptoms and Problems of Deficiency |
|---|---|---|---|
| MAGNESIUM | An important nutrient for 300 biochemical reactions in the body; benefits muscle/nerve function, heart rhythm, immune system, strong bones; regulates calcium, copper, zinc, potassium, vitamin D levels | Green vegetables, peas | Changes in appetite, nausea, vomiting, fatigue, cramps, numbness, tingling, seizures, heart spasms, personality changes, abnormal heart rhythm |
| ALPHA LIPOIC ACID | Increases energy, blood flow to nerves, glutathione levels in brain, insulin sensitivity, effectiveness of vitamins C and E, other antioxidants | Spinach, broccoli | Diabetic neuropathy, reduced muscle mass, atherosclerosis, Alzheimer's disease, failure to thrive, brain atrophy, high lactic acid |
| COPPER | Benefits bone formation; involved in healing process, energy production, hair and skin coloring, taste sensitivity; stimulates iron absorption; helps metabolize several fatty acids | Dark leafy greens | Osteoporosis, anemia, baldness, diarrhea, general weakness, impaired respiratory function, myelopathy, decreased skin pigment, reduced resistance to infection |

| Nutrient | What It Does/ Body Systems It Benefits | Green and Other Vegetable Sources | Symptoms and Problems of Deficiency |
|---|---|---|---|
| VITAMIN B2 | Helps regulate metabolism and helps with carbohydrate conversion; breaks down fats and protein; benefits digestion, nervous system, skin, hair, eyes, mouth, liver | Mushrooms, green vegetables | Anemia, decreased free radical protection, cataracts, poor thyroid function, vitamin B6 deficiency, fatigue, elevated homocysteine levels |
| FOLATE | Boosts mental health, infant DNA/RNA; works with vitamin B12 to regulate red blood cell production, iron function; reduces homocysteine levels; is especially important during pregnancy for the growth of the baby and later for the growth of adolescents | Tomato juice, green vegetables | Anemia, issues with immune function, fatigue, insomnia, hair, high homocysteine levels, cardiovascular disease |
| VITAMIN A | Eyes, immune function, skin, essential cell growth and development | Orange or green vegetables | Night blindness, issues with immune function, zinc deficiency, fat malabsorption |
| VITAMIN K | Aids in the formation of clotting factors and bone proteins and the formation of glucose into glycogen for storage in the liver | Kale, turnip greens, spinach, broccoli, lettuce, cabbage, asparagus, watercress, peas | Excessive bleeding, a history of bruising, appearance of ruptured capillaries or menorrhagia (heavy periods) |

Incorporating more vegetables into your diet will also help curb your appetite for unhealthy foods. Many of us turn to sweets, simple carbohydrates and processed food because they are easy or we crave them or find comfort in them. Unfortunately, the more of these foods we consume, the more we want them. Not only can this introduce toxic chemicals into the body, but it will also raise blood sugar levels, possibly leading down a path toward diabetes or insulin resistance.

Despite the overwhelming evidence of vegetables' profound benefits on our health, they are conspicuously lacking in most of our modern diets. Relatively few of us are getting that amount that I recommend, which is five to nine servings a day. (Figure that each serving is about the size of the palm of your hand.) As a society we are overfed but undernourished. But adding greens to your diet doesn't have to be difficult or expensive or mean a sacrifice in taste.

Thankfully, organic veggies are also increasingly available. Eating organic is important because it reduces your exposure to pesticides, toxins that can kill off the good bacteria that are necessary for healthy digestion. The good news is that in addition to local farmers' markets and health food stores, more and more supermarkets are including organic options in their produce sections. According to a national 2009 study cosponsored by the Organic Trade Association, nearly three-quarters (73 percent) of U.S. families buy organic products at least occasionally, chiefly for health reasons. This is an encouraging trend.

## The Many Varieties of Green

When many people hear "green leafy vegetables," they think of iceberg lettuce. Unfortunately, the pale, genetically engineered lettuce we are usually served in restaurants just doesn't have the power-packed nutrition of other types of greens. Broccoli is a popular favorite and is commonly available. Green cabbage is excellent raw or as sauerkraut. You can choose among bok choy, napa cabbage, kale, collards, watercress, mustard greens, broccoli, rabe, dandelion and other leafy greens for your salads and recipes. Arugula, endive, chicory, lettuce and wild greens are generally consumed raw but can be eaten in any creative way that tastes good to you.

To begin, especially if your head is swimming as a result of all these unfamiliar names, buy some mixed greens and try adding something new a little bit at a time. One week, experiment with arugula in your mixed greens. Another week, try endive. The next week sample mustard greens. This way you can try something new mixed with something familiar and make changes easily and gradually.

Certain greens, such as spinach, Swiss chard and beet greens, should be eaten only in moderation because they are high in oxalic acid, which can deplete your calcium levels. An easy way to balance this effect is to cook these greens with a food with a high fat content, like tofu, seeds, nuts, beans, butter or other animal fat, or oil.

## Cooking Tips

Speaking of cooking your greens, there are a variety of methods to try: steaming, blanching, sautéing, even lightly pickling, as in a pressed salad. Blanching is a culinary word for boiling, and this method produces greens that are plump and relaxed. Be sure to get the water boiling first and then add your greens. Cook them for only 30 to 45 seconds so that the nutrients stay in the greens and do not move out into the water. If you're blanching organic greens, an added health benefit is that you can drink the cooking water as a broth or a tea, or add it to whatever else you're cooking if the recipe calls for additional liquid. Steaming makes greens more fibrous and tight. And of course, the familiar raw green salad is a refreshing way to eat greens while supplying healthy live enzymes.

Don't forget to wash your veggies before cooking them or eating them raw. Even organic foods should be washed. A good way to wash greens is to fill a *clean* sink with cold water and add two tablespoons of white vinegar. You won't taste the vinegar, but it will naturally disinfect any germs. Let leafy greens soak for three minutes, rinse and then resoak in clean water for another three minutes. Dry your greens by putting them through a salad spinner before you use or store them. For all other vegetables and fruit with a skin (such as eggplant, oranges or lemons), soak them in the vinegar water described above for 20 minutes, rinse them and resoak in clean water for another 20 minutes, and dry before you store or use them.

For a super-quick, fun and easy way to get your fruits and veggies, try a green smoothie: Just blend two cups of water, two to four servings of fruit, and five ounces of greens with ice. If you use unsweetened frozen fruit, you can forgo the ice. Banana, mango and spinach or banana, raspberry and spinach might be a good combination to try initially. Keep experimenting until you find combinations that you enjoy. If the only thing you do after reading this chapter is add one green smoothie to your diet every day, you'll have significantly enhanced your wellness!

Below are a few recipes to get you started incorporating more greens into your diet. A food processor is most helpful for many of these recipes, but you can chop and dice veggies and greens with a knife or an inexpensive "chopper" hand tool instead. I also recommend using a salad spinner to dry your greens, but to reduce your costs, use a paper towel to remove most moisture and let the rest air-dry. To create the green smoothies, you will need to buy a blender, which you can find for as little as $20.

According to the Institute for Integrative Nutrition, when we eat food whole, some 80 percent of the nutrients go right out our back end, so a food processor is a great tool for breaking down the cellular membrane of vegetables in order to get more nutrients from them

**Cherry Bomb Smoothie**

2 cups water
Half of 10-ounce package frozen cherries (pitted)
1 clementine
1 apple
1 banana
Half of 1 bunch kale
1 tablespoon flaxseed, ground

Put all ingredients in a high-power blender and blend until smooth.

### Raspberry-Pear Green Smoothie

2 cups water
1 fresh pear
Half of 10-ounce bag frozen raspberries
1 banana
1 orange
1 tablespoon soaked chia seeds
3–4 collard greens

Put all ingredients in a high-power blender and blend until smooth.

### Blueberry and Peach Green Smoothie

2 cups water
10-ounce bag frozen blueberries
1 fresh peach
1 banana
1 pitted date
1–2 heads bok choy
1 tablespoon unhulled sesame seeds

Put all ingredients in a high-power blender and blend until smooth.

### Blended Green Vegetable Soup

2–3 cups fresh green beans, trimmed
2–3 zucchini, cut into thirds
2–3 celery stalks, cut into fourths
1/2 bunch asparagus
4–8 kale leaves
1/2 bunch parsley

1–2 cloves garlic

Steam the green beans, zucchini, celery, asparagus and kale over water until soft but still green. Remove the vegetables from the water, but don't discard the water just yet. Place the cooked vegetables, plus the parsley and garlic, in a blender and puree until smooth. Add a bit of the steaming water as needed to thin. Season to taste with minced ginger, cayenne, turmeric or other herbs.

**Veg Shred**
Include a handful of any of the following vegetables:
Kale
Swiss chard
Collard greens
Dandelion greens
Beets
Beet greens
Broccoli
Cauliflower
Carrots
Celery
Cabbage (red or green)
Parsley
Radish (any variety)
Turnip

This recipe can be made to fit your tastes. If you are new to veggies, try it with a couple of your favorites and then add a new veggie each time you make it. You can use three or four of the listed veggies or all of them. The taste will change every time you make it, depending on the ingredients and amounts you use.

Dry the greens in a salad spinner or with a paper towel and let them air dry. (It is important that the veggies are dry before you begin to process them.) Using a seven-cup food processor, attach the chopping blade and chop all the leafy greens. You may have to do this in batches. Put the chopped greens in a bowl and change the blade to a grater. One by one, feed all of the other vegetables through the processor's chute until finished. Add these vegetables to the bowl and mix with the greens.

Store the finished Veg Shred in an airtight container (glass or stainless steel). It will keep fresh in the refrigerator for up to five days. Save "wet" veggies (such as tomatoes, zucchini or cucumbers) as toppers; do not include them in the mix because they will make the Veg Shred soggy, and it won't keep as long.

When you're ready to eat the Veg Shred, get creative. Pull out one to two cups of the mix and top it with beans, goat cheese, tomatoes, sprouts, nuts, seeds, dried cranberries, raisins—whatever strikes your fancy—and the dressing of your choice. You can also toss the Veg Shred in with eggs to make a power-packed omelet; or try adding it to soup or a stir-fry. Have fun with it!

## Personal Stories

Angela Rizzo was overweight, perimenopausal and had suffered with migraines for years. Then she began experiencing visual and speech problems, which doctors sometimes consider to be "ministroke" symptoms. Tests also indicated that she was showing signs of the possible onset of multiple sclerosis. She saw a neurologist, who suggested an antidepressant used to help prevent migraines, but Angela was uneasy about taking the medicine because of potential side effects of weight gain and an increased—ironic—chance of depression, among others.

As Angela reflected about what to do, her inner voice encouraged her to see me. She filled out a detailed survey so that we could look at her lifestyle as well as her symptoms. She was already keeping a food diary, which was very helpful. Her blood work revealed high blood-sugar levels, and our neurological chiropractor at YWC determined that Angela was unknowingly eating far too much sugar by consuming a lot of fruit and large quantities of what she thought was "healthy" cereal, without the correct balance of protein. Angela learned a key truth—that she could eat good food, or food that is marketed as good (sometimes these are not the same!), but if she did not eat it in the proper balance for her body, it would not contribute to her wellness.

As a result of my practice's collaboration with her, Angela decided to change her diet and her life. She cut out all "white" food, meaning she ate no processed food, no white rice, no potatoes, no sugar and no flour. She also stopped drinking alcohol, and she stopped drinking diet soda pop after learning that diet drinks not only can cause water retention but can also increase carbohydrate cravings. She began eating five or six small, well-balanced meals each day, adding protein in the form of chicken, turkey, eggs, beans, nuts and fish. She began going on walks with her partner and her dog for at least 30 minutes every evening.

After two weeks of diet and lifestyle change, Angela was losing weight and starting to feel better. She eventually lost 16 pounds. Her headaches disappeared, as did her hot flashes. It seemed like a miracle! But it wasn't a miracle at all. It was a completely natural phenomenon. When you give the body the nutrition and support it needs, it can heal a wide variety of diseases.

Angela says, "People talk about 'middle-age weight gain' like it's an inevitable fact of life, but it's not. You control it. Getting control of your diet is the most significant change you can make, for your weight and your overall health. And it really *is* all in your mind. You tell yourself that you have to do this, that you are in control, that you can be better. Then you do it. You make the commitment to yourself and you do it."

Nowadays, Angela drinks lots of water as well as some types of tea, but she passes on coffee. She watches her portion size, and she refuses to have unhealthy food in the house (for those times when she might be tempted to make a less-than-healthy choice). Angela avoids fast food and vending machines, saying, "Why would I put that poison in my body again?" She feels great. She looks great. She has lots of energy for all the things she's doing and enjoying in her life. And even if she occasionally suffers through stressful times in other areas of her life, she's able to function well and handle the stress because her overall health is good. When asked about the lifestyle choices she makes, Angela says, "Life is short; I really want to enjoy it! Living this way, I can."

Another client, Eddie Penrice, came to my practice because he had a back injury that did not heal and he was in constant pain. To compound his health situation, he was taking medicine to treat a variety of other issues, including diabetes, high blood pressure and high cholesterol. Initially Eddie came to see me for acupuncture treatments, which gave him some relief.

He decided to try adding chiropractic treatments, so we took the standard X-rays of his spine. Upon seeing his X-rays, Eddie was appalled. As is common in the United States in this day and age, his intestines were full of undigested matter, probably 20 pounds or more.

Eddie had heard the phrase, "Death begins in the colon," and after seeing those X-rays, he believed that he was seeing how that could be—and probably was—true in his own body. He decided right then that he would clean out his colon and not put any more substances in his body that could end up sitting and rotting in his intestines.

Eddie began a 100 percent raw diet, meaning he ate no meat, no dairy and no cooked food. He was already taking nutritional supplements for his disease, and listening to his own inner guidance, he decided to stop all his medications and let his body utilize the food he gave it in order to see whether he could heal naturally.

Eddie says, "After two weeks, it was like I had walked through a door, and there was no way I could go back. I had strength, energy, a completely different physical feeling … a powerful feeling! I realized that cooked food is just the shell of food, not food itself. I learned how to eat to live, not live to eat, as most people do. It was like a 'born again' experience— that powerful, that profound an awakening to my consciousness."

Before his diet change, Eddie ate meat, dairy, cooked food, fast food, sweets, cakes, ice cream and home-cooked "soul" food. Now he starts his day with 20 ounces of fresh water in the morning. After 45 minutes, he eats fruit or fresh juice or gluten-free cereal with almond milk for breakfast. Eddie munches on a salad all day long. He drinks no caffeine. He takes a daily probiotic, which is a nutritional supplement of healthy intestinal flora. He always has plenty of water, nuts and fruit available, and he never lets himself get really hungry. Therefore, he is never tempted to eat something unhealthy.

Within 30 to 45 days of changing his diet, Eddie had lost 30 pounds. He did this with very little exercise, which was restricted because of his back injury. His bowel movements also changed. Eddie will tell you that they are a "pleasant" experience now—no straining, no discomfort and no foul odor like before.

He states, "If people would embrace themselves, not embrace the forces that say 'You cannot,' they would realize that embracing the positive is just as easy as embracing the negative. If you embrace the positive things you need to do for yourself, you'll be amazed. When we ingest what God gave us to ingest, our bodies work! Ever since I was a little kid, I would pray, 'God, I want to be able to live to 100 years old!' I've now changed that prayer to say, 'God, I want to be able to live to at least 100 years old, in my right mind, with a strong body, able to do and help anybody that needs my help.' And with God's help, I know I can do it. We all can. First we have to have a desire to get out of our circumstance of food-related illness. To say, 'I *am* sick of being sick. I *will* make the changes.' And then you *do* make the changes. Then you *have* the life you want. I am, I will, I do, I have ... The power comes from within."

## Practical Tips for Your Journey

1. If you are ready, begin your diet change with just one thing: Invest in a good blender if you can (but any blender on the market can handle the recipes in this book if the veggies are cut up), and start by adding a delicious green smoothie each day.

2. Once you've mastered adding the smoothie, for a second easy change, sauté a veggie each night to add to your dinner.

3. Consider investing in a food processor, and start to create your Veg Shred, which makes a great salad or side dish. Prepare enough to eat for several days. Add wet veggies like cucumber, peppers and zucchini just before you eat the Veg Shred. Add other ingredients according to your tastes.

4. Try this strategy that we at YWC teach our wellness and nutrition clients: Shop for the week on Saturday and then prepare large batches of food on Sunday and again on Wednesday. You can make a large portion and eat from it for several days. You do lose some nutrients as fresh food sits in the refrigerator, so it's preferable to prepare each meal each day. But since that isn't always possible, preparing batches twice a week is a good compromise.

5. Aim for a one-to-one ratio of raw to cooked greens in your diet.

## Your Space

Use this page to make notes and write your own reflections on going for the greens.

_____

_____

_____

_____

_____

_____

_____

_____

_____

_____

_____

_____

_____

_____

# Chapter 6

# Eat From the Sea—And Enjoy the Sun!

Nature provides everything we need to be healthy in mind, body and spirit. In this chapter I discuss two of those gifts: fatty acids—in particular omega-3s, abundant in fish oils—and vitamin D, which is available from the sun. Both nutrients support your organs and organ systems at the cellular level. You can't get much more basic and critical than that! When cells—all types of cells—are not functioning properly, just about everything in the body is affected. Before you learn more about why and how to incorporate omega-3s and vitamin D into your life, ask yourself if you suffer from any of the problems mentioned in the questions below. If you do, getting more of one or both nutrients might make a difference.

## Questions to Consider

- Do you have a weak immune system?
- Are your bones weak?
- Do you have itchy skin?
- Are you often agitated, easily upset or nervous?
- Is it difficult for you to concentrate?
- Does your mind feel sluggish?
- Do you suffer from depression or anxiety?
- Do you struggle with forgetfulness?
- Are you finding it difficult to get motivated?
- Is your vision blurry?
- Do you crave sweets during the day?

ॐ Do you experience headaches in the afternoon?

ॐ Do you have joint pain?

ॐ Do you have inflammation in any area of your body?

ॐ Has your doctor told you that your HDL (high-density lipoproteins) levels are low?

## The Power of Seafood

"The concept of total wellness recognizes that our every thought, word and behavior affects our greater health and well-being. And we, in turn, are affected not only emotionally but also physically and spiritually."

—Greg Anderson

Each cell in our bodies is surrounded by a membrane made up primarily of fatty acids. This membrane allows the proper amounts of nutrients to enter the cell, and it ensures that waste products are efficiently removed. For a cell to work properly, to hold water and vital nutrients, to protect us from nonstop bombardment of free-radical damage and to communicate effectively with other cells, its membrane has to be healthy and fluid.

Because cell membranes are composed of fat, the quality of our cell membranes is directly related to the quality and amount of good fat we eat. When we eat a lot of saturated fats, which are solid at room temperature, the result is cell membranes that are hard and lack fluidity. Eating a diet rich in unsaturated fats that are liquid at room temperature produces cell membranes with a high degree of fluidity, and this promotes wellness in every organ and every organ system of our bodies.

Unsaturated fats, however, are not all the same, and they are not all good for us. In order to produce a product with a higher melting point (good for cooking) and a longer shelf life (good for storage), food manufacturers add hydrogen atoms to unsaturated fats (a process called hydrogenation), making them more saturated (saturated fats are "saturated" with hydrogen atoms). In this process, however, a type of unsaturated fat called a trans fat is created. Trans fats are simply unsaturated fats that have undergone hydrogenation but have not been fully converted to saturated fats. Trans fats are not essential, and they do not promote good health. In fact, trans fats increase our risk of heart disease, and we absolutely need to avoid them!

Two other types of unsaturated fats are monounsaturated and polyunsaturated fats, and their names derive from their molecular structures. Both are nutritionally important. Monounsaturated fats (like olive oil) are liquid at room temperature but harden when refrigerated. Polyunsaturated fats (like soybean oil) are also liquid at room temperature and remain liquid when refrigerated or put in the freezer. Both unsaturated fats are different from the saturated fats we are familiar with, like butter and cheese, which are solid when refrigerated and remain solid at room temperature.

You've probably been hearing a lot lately about one particular type of polyunsaturated fat: omega-3 fatty acids. That's because we're learning more and more about why these healthy fats are profoundly important for wellness. They are one of two fatty acids that have been called essential because the body must have them to survive. The body cannot manufacture these fatty acids on its own so we must eat them in our food or take supplements.

There are three types of omega-3 fatty acids: EPA (eicosapentaenoic acid) and DHA (docosahexaenoic acid) are found in cold-water fish such as salmon, tuna, halibut, herring and mackerel. The only plant food that contains much EPA or DHA is fresh seaweed. The third type of omega-3 is ALA (alpha-linolenic acid). Its dietary sources include flaxseed oil, dark green leafy vegetables, some vegetable oils and avocados, walnuts and hemp seeds.

The first two are the more critical of the omega-3 fatty acids—your heart and brain need DHA and EPA. ALA is also important, but if your intake of omega-3s is just from ALA sources, then your body may not be getting the full benefits of these fatty acids. While your body can convert ALA into DHA and EPA, this will happen only if all of your organs and systems are functioning at optimal levels. Even if your body is in excellent condition, you will likely only be able to convert up to 20 percent of ALA to DHA and EPA. The only way to ensure that you get the proper amounts of these two important omega-3s is to consume fish oil (taking fish oil supplements or eating the types of fish described above).

So what's so great about omega-3? There is considerable evidence that adding it to your daily diet in the form of fish oil has a significant impact on neurological disorders, mental illness, including depression, heart health, and inflammation. The scientific support is such that the FDA has even approved an omega-3 pill as medicine.[1] Here are some specific ways that it can benefit your body:

§ Keeping your cell membranes fluid.

§ Improving your immune system.

§ Reducing inflammation in all areas of your body.

§ Keeping your blood from clotting excessively.

§ Balancing the amount of cholesterol and triglycerides in your blood.

§ Stopping the thickening of your arteries.

§ Causing your arteries to dilate and relax.

§ Reducing your risk of obesity.

§ Improving your ability to respond to insulin and manage blood sugar.

§ Helping prevent the growth of cancer.

§ Reducing depression and anxiety.

§ Supporting the health of your gastrointestinal tract.

§ Improving the health of your skin.

Omega-6 is the other essential fatty acid. At his Web site, Andrew Weil, M.D., explains that omega-6 is important because it helps construct hormones that "increase inflammation (an important component of the immune response), blood clotting and cell proliferation."[2] Dietary sources of omega-6 include nuts, seeds, and corn, safflower, sunflower, soybean and canola oils. An easy way to remember this is that omega-3 is found in green things, and in things that *eat* green things—like fish and grass-fed beef, for example—while omega-6 is found in grains, nuts and seeds.

My colleague Corey Priest, D.C., is a specialist in functional medicine, a branch of medicine that looks at the person as a whole—at the person's structural, neurological, physio-logical and emotional components—and not simply at individual systems. His main focus is physiology (the chemistry of the body). Dr. Priest explains the importance of balance in our consumption of omega-3 and omega-6: "The appropriate ratio of omega-6 to omega-3 in human blood is two omega-6 for every one omega-3. But the average American eating the standard American diet has a blood ratio of 26 omega-6 for every one omega-3, at best. This imbalance can lead to a variety of inflammatory diseases, including depression and anxiety, cardiovascular disease, type 2 diabetes, fatigue, dry and itchy skin, brittle hair and nails, inability to concentrate, constipation, frequent colds, lack of physical endurance and joint pain."

It makes sense that your risk of developing the following health conditions could be greatly diminished if you added the recommended amounts of omega-3 to your diet in the proper balance to omega-6:

- Alzheimer's disease
- Asthma
- Attention-deficit/hyperactivity disorder (ADHD)
- Autism
- Bipolar disorder
- Cancer
- Cardiovascular disease
- Depression
- Diabetes
- Eczema

- § High blood pressure
- § Huntington's disease
- § Lupus
- § Migraine headaches
- § Multiple sclerosis
- § Obesity
- § Osteoarthritis
- § Osteoporosis
- § Psoriasis
- § Rheumatoid arthritis

**A word of caution:** There are some conditions that need careful monitoring when you're adding omega-3 to your diet. People who have disorders involving bleeding, who bruise very easily or who are taking blood thinners—as well as people taking prescription blood pressure medications and/or anticoagulants—need to consult with a medical practitioner before taking supplemental omega-3 fatty acids. As with most things, moderation is important. The FDA recommends no more than three grams of EPA and DHA per day, with no more than two grams coming from a dietary supplement.

When you add new foods or supplements to your diet, it is important to remember that the body uses nutrition to repair itself on a cellular level, so it can take months to experience symptom relief as your body rebuilds and restores your organs and organ systems from the cellular level up. Stay the course, and be patient!

## The Power of a Sun Vitamin

Osteoporosis, multiple sclerosis, high blood pressure, diabetes and cancer are all wreaking havoc in our society. Some of them, such as osteoporosis, are especially devastating to women. One part of the arsenal we can use to fight them is simple and readily available: vitamin D.

Vitamin D has rightfully gained its recent popularity among medical specialists and wellness experts. As modern research explains, the benefits of adequate levels of vitamin D go far beyond helping bones stay strong and curing rickets in children. This vital nutrient has an effect on every major system in the body, including hormones.

I have mentioned in other chapters the importance of blood-sugar regulation and its dramatic effects on overall health. The body is made up of trillions of cells, and vitamin D is responsible for regulating those cells. Because vitamin D regulates cells throughout the body, it can significantly influence insulin regulation (blood-sugar regulation) and immune function, as well as help prevent inflammation and cancer.

Studies show that vitamin D deficiency appears to be very common, with men, women, children and infants lacking adequate levels. (An inexpensive blood test can determine your levels.) This comes as no surprise, since we spend more time indoors than ever before, and the main source of vitamin D is sunshine. Human beings can produce vitamin D3 in the skin through exposure to ultraviolet B (UVB) radiation from sunlight.

Because of the rise in skin cancers over the last 25 years or so, however, we are encouraged to slather on sunscreen. According to Michael F. Holick, M.D., Ph.D., of the Boston

⌒

University School of Medicine, a sunblock with an SPF of 8 reduces the skin's vitamin D production by 95 percent. But the National Institutes of Health report that as little as 10 to 15 minutes of sun exposure at least three days a week (without sunscreen) may be enough to prevent deficiencies.[3] In Chapter 1, I encouraged you to reap the benefits of vitamin D when I recommended walking in nature to relax and rejuvenate; just be sure to soak up your daily dose of sunshine before applying whatever sunscreen you choose to use.

Vitamin D can also be obtained from diet. Foods naturally rich in it include salmon and mackerel (note that they are also good sources of DHA and EPA omega-3); sardines, tuna, eggs and liver are also good sources. Foods fortified with vitamin D can help you meet the daily requirements established by the federal government: 200 international units (IUs) for 19- to 50-year-olds, 400 IUs for adults 51 to 70, and 600 IUs for those 71 years and older. But keep in mind that foods fortified with vitamin D are chemically altered to add a nutrient not naturally found in them.

People for whom sunshine and diet alone may not suffice can maintain adequate levels of vitamin D by taking supplements. Some experts recommend a vitamin D daily intake of 800 to 1,000 IUs, and recommendations vary for people who are dark-skinned or spend little time outdoors. Ask your doctor to test your vitamin D levels before you add this supplement to your diet. And as with any supplement, be sure to read the labels carefully. D3, found naturally in the body and available in a supplement, is more effective than D2.

## Personal Stories

Linda Pfingsten is a client in her 50s who has a family history of high cholesterol, and she was concerned about her own cholesterol levels. She also suffered from continual joint pain. Initially she came to see me for relief from that pain and from lower back pain. She was already taking omega-3 fatty acids in pill form. Over time, we worked together on the mechanical and lifestyle components affecting her pain level.

I also suggested that she make a change in her supplements, switching from her pills to a higher-dose liquid product. At first Linda resisted the idea. She was used to taking what she had always taken, and she didn't really believe that there was a big difference in the quality of one brand over another. However, as we discussed the need of the body for variety and the benefits of taking a supplement of truly excellent quality, she opened herself to the idea of trying my suggestion for 30 to 90 days. She began taking 1,700 mg of liquid omega-3s two times a day. Today her joint pain is significantly decreased, and her cholesterol levels are excellent. Linda was so pleased by the results that when her daughter, who has survived cancer, was directed by both her medical doctor and her cancer specialist to take omega-3 supplements as a preventive measure, Linda made sure her daughter got the highest-quality omega-3s available.

Linda reports that in addition to her improved cholesterol levels and decreased pain, she no longer seems to deal with the everyday viruses and bacterial illnesses that affect so many people around her. She encourages others to research what else is out there, to be open to trying something new, to give your body the best nutrients available and to advocate for your own wellness. Linda will be the first to tell you that if one doctor or other medical professional is not able to help you address your problem, you need to keep looking until you find someone who will.

Lee Harris, a client I mentioned in Chapter 3, takes a high daily dose—10,000 mg—of omega-3 fatty acids. He has been able to discontinue his cholesterol medication altogether, a fact that he attributes to the high dosage of omega-3. In addition, Lee's triglyceride levels are very good, and he is experiencing a new level of vitality in his life.

Another client, Rachel Lincoln, was in her early 50s when she came in for treatment of severe perimenopausal symptoms. She was having extreme hot flashes, anxiety and depression. Traditional medicines were not alleviating her symptoms, and they were even causing her to gain weight. Her solution was to stop taking them altogether. Nothing was helping, and she was miserable!

Rachel began working with my colleague Corey Priest, and they focused on making healthy diet changes. Within *one week* of adding 6,000 mg of omega-3s to her daily diet, Rachel called to report that all her hot flashes were gone (and, as it turned out, never to return), and her anxiety and depression had lifted significantly. Omega-3 fatty acids, happily, did not cause her to gain any weight. She was beyond excited, feeling better than she had in a long time—and Corey and I were just as excited as she was! While most people don't respond as quickly as Rachel did, every once in a while we see these dramatic and inspiring results. Every time one of our patients triumphs as a result of the work that we do together, we share in that person's joy and celebration.

~

Francene Lisle, 57, is a dear client and proud Texan. She became a patient in 1999 but moved back to Texas in 2004. In 2005 she began to notice a significant decrease in her energy level and an increase in the frequency of upper respiratory infections that never seemed to end entirely. She went to countless doctors, who diagnosed her with fatigue and sinus infections. She was on round after round of antibiotics and steroids. In 2007 Francene's family suffered a terrible loss when her daughter, grandchild and son-in-law were in a traffic accident; her son-in-law did not survive. The stress and sadness caused her health to decline further; now she was also having difficulty sleeping and suffered from depression.

Francene traveled to see a friend in Kansas City that year. While she was in town, she called me. After hearing her story and her symptoms since I had last seen her, I suggested she go through a detoxifying regimen and then add in considerable amounts of omega-3 fatty acids (in the form of fish oil) to her diet. She felt better after the detox, but admitted that she had not consistently been taking the omega-3s.

In 2008 Francene moved back to Kansas City and began seeing me regularly. She began to pay more attention to taking the omega-3s, and we added acupuncture to her treatment. Although she was improving, something was still not there. I referred her to a physician, Rebecca Gernon, who I knew had a holistic approach. After a physical, including blood work, it was determined that Francene was seriously deficient in vitamin D. Her D level was a 9, when minimum normal levels are around 32. Francene began taking 50,000 IUs of D3 a week for eight weeks, followed by a maintenance dose of 5,000 IUs daily. Follow-up testing showed a D level of 34.

~

Francene's upper respiratory infections stopped, she began sleeping through the night, she regained her energy and began exercising, her depression disappeared, and even her cholesterol level dropped dramatically. To this day, Francene faithfully keeps omega-3s and vitamin D a part of her daily regimen. She will tell you that if she runs out of either one and doesn't take it for a few days, she immediately feels the difference in her body. Francene has said, "If I ever have to move away again, I'll travel back to Kansas City frequently to continue seeing Dr. Robin." And I am grateful to have made a difference in her life. That's my life's mission!

## Practical Tips for Your Journey

1. In order for omega-3s to function optimally in your body, make sure your diet includes a sufficient amount of vitamin B6, vitamin B3, vitamin C, magnesium and zinc. There are also certain amino acids that aid in the absorption, utilization and functionality of omega-3 fatty acids, so it is a good idea to discuss your diet with a nutritional professional when and if you have questions or concerns. In addition, make sure you limit your intake of saturated fat and trans fat.

2. When you purchase an omega-3 supplement—available as soft gels or bottled liquids—remember that these oils are extremely susceptible to damage from oxygen, heat and light. When exposed to these elements for too long, the fatty acids in the oil become rancid. Rancidity not only tastes and smells bad, it also reduces the nutritional value of the fatty acids and produces free radicals, which play a role in various forms of disease. Choose a certified-organic

product that has been refrigerated and is packaged in a dark brown or green glass jar if it is a liquid. Be sure to store the liquid product in your refrigerator or freezer once you open it. Also check the ingredients list to make sure there is no filler oil, especially no soybean oil.

3. Make sure your supplement also contains the powerful antioxidant vitamin E, which is added to the oil to prevent the fatty acids from becoming oxidized (rancid). It should be indicated on the label or referenced at the manufacturer's Web site. Your supplement should never taste "fishy" or smell bad.

4. Look for a ratio of 18 EPA to 12 DHA, because this is how those omega-3 fatty acids occur in nature.

5. Make sure your supplement is tested (assayed) by a third party to ensure that it is free from toxins and heavy metals and that the ingredients inside the bottle or capsule are the same as what the label claims. Reputable manufacturers of supplements will either indicate on their label or Web site that the contents have been certified pure. If you are purchasing from your chiropractor or a health food store, either source may also have research or materials that indicate the purity.

6. Get a good physical and have your vitamin D levels checked.

7. Consider taking vitamin D supplements, especially if you live in states north of Oklahoma, from October to May.

8. Doctor's orders: Get outside and play, and soak up some of Mother Nature's medicine. And don't forget to do the same thing with, and for, your kids!

## Your Space

Use this page to make notes and write your own reflections on eating from the sea and enjoying the sun.

# Chapter 7

# Drink to Your Health

Water is similar to breathing in that we cannot survive long without it. Fundamental to all life, water is required for all of our bodily functions down to the cellular level. It also cleanses and purifies our bodies, literally inside and out—even spiritually for many faiths. I promise you that if you incorporate the healthy habit of drinking sufficient water into your life, you will feel a wave of renewed health wash over you. Could you be dehydrated? (Consuming fluids is not the same thing as drinking water.) Your answers to the following questions might tell the tale.

## Questions to Consider

- Do you have any skin conditions?
- Do you have allergies?
- Are you tired and lethargic?
- Do you often feel flushed?
- Do you have asthma?
- Are you irritable, anxious, dejected or depressed?
- Do you suffer from frequent headaches or back pain?
- Do you find it hard to concentrate?
- When you pull your skin away from the bone, does it return quickly to its original form?
- Do you wake up stiff and aching?
- Do you have high blood pressure?

ᕗ Are you constipated?

ᕗ Do you suffer from irresistible food cravings?

ᕗ Do you urinate at least five times a day?

ᕗ Are you dealing with an autoimmune disorder or arthritis?

ᕗ Do you have type 2 diabetes?

ᕗ Do you drink enough water every day? (For example, if you weigh 150 pounds, do you drink at least 75 ounces of water each day?)

---

### The Power of Water

"Water is life's matter and matrix, mother and medium. There is no life without water."

—Albert Szent-Gyorgyi

"Water is the only drink for a wise man."

—Henry David Thoreau

---

The final wellness practice in this book is one that I've already mentioned, and very likely something you've heard many times: Drink more water! Water is involved in the body's essential processes, including but not limited to bringing nutrients and oxygen to cells; removing waste products, free radicals and toxins from cells; cushioning bones; lubricating joints; maintaining the body's basal metabolic rate and cells' electrical conductivity; growing and repairing cells and tissues; regulating body temperature; maintaining DNA structure and function; and supporting the immune system and digestive processes.

When fully hydrated, our bodies are almost 80 percent water. This water must be replaced every day. Sedentary people regularly lose significant water through evaporation and perspiration, and active people lose much more. Water loss has immediate effects in our bodies. A study of athletes cited by John Douillard, Ph.D., in his 2003 book *Perfect Health for Kids* showed that if athletes lost even 2 percent of their body weight through water loss during exercise, they would experience a 25 percent decrease in strength and athletic performance.[1] That's quite significant! He recommends weighing yourself before and after exercise and then drinking 16 ounces of water for every pound lost during the workout. This is important for children as well as adults.

Chemically, water is made up of two hydrogen atoms with one oxygen atom. It is a polar molecule, which means it has a slight electrical charge that attracts other substances to it. Water, on a molecular level, is "sticky" by nature. Other polar substances include alcohol, food flavorings, salts, sugars and vinegar. When you put these in water, they dissolve. Oils, on the other hand, are nonpolar; they have no electrical charge. They do not dissolve in water; in fact, they do not mix at all.

Because a water molecule is sticky, it attracts anything with an electrical charge. This is why we can mix things like instant tea and lemonade with water. This stickiness is also what makes water a solvent beyond compare for the various substances that are absorbed by our bodies, such as enzymes, hormones, electrolytes and nutrients. Water's stickiness, however, can also cause problems. In *Perfect Health for Kids*,

Dr. Douillard explains that water passes in and out of our cells via specialized channels called aquaporins. But when the water molecules have materials stuck to them, they become too large to fit through the aquaporins and cannot get into our cells. It's like trying to crawl through a very small tunnel with 15 large backpacks attached to your body— impossible!

Some of the molecules that get stuck to the water we drink come from contamination—natural or man-made. This can occur naturally from volcanoes, storms and earthquakes. Most often, however, water is contaminated by human beings through factory by-products, plant fertilizers, leaks in underground tanks and sewers, pesticides and pharmaceuticals (those that aren't metabolized by the body and are therefore excreted in urine, as well as drugs thrown in the trash or down the drain).

I have had a number of clients tell me that they are not dehydrated because they drink cola, pop or some other beverage all day. But as I said at the beginning of this chapter, consuming fluid does not equal hydration. It's very important to drink water with nothing added (no diet-drink flavorings, no minerals and no fruit juice). Unfortunately, most of the water we drink is saturated with dissolved solids like sugars, minerals, food coloring or other chemicals or contaminants. F. Batmanghelidj, M.D., explains in *Water for Health, for Healing, for Life*, that although beverages with these substances are not dehydrating like alcohol, caffeinated tea or coffee, which are diuretics, they do not actually contribute to the water our bodies need because they flow right *over* our cells and cannot get *into* our cells through the aquaporins.[2]

It's why people can drink lots and lots of fluids and still feel thirsty—the fluid really is passing right through them.

I realize that much of the medical establishment will tell you that fluid is fluid and all of them hydrate equally. There are experts and science that support both perspectives. However, it would be difficult to find anyone who would say that straight-up water is not still the best option. I have witnessed time and time again in my practice the unparalleled positive impact when clients don't just add water to their regimen but replace all other fluids with water.

Another good habit to practice is drinking your water at room temperature. Cold water contracts the esophagus and the stomach, and this makes it much harder for your body to absorb the fluid. If you have traveled to Europe, you know that when you order water, you are brought room-temperature water with no ice. Ice water is an American custom. In this case, we would do well to emulate our friends overseas.

## Water: The Ultimate Waste Remover

Let's consider how water is related to asthma and allergies. When our bodies get dehydrated, our mucous membranes are unable to stay moist. This triggers a histamine response, and we get excess mucus in our sinuses and in our digestive tracts. We get swelling and edema in our lungs and bronchial tubes, leading to shortness of breath, the first sign of an asthma attack. Simple, adequate hydration can greatly contribute to reduced asthmatic incidents.

Dehydration also makes it impossible for our bodies' lymphatic systems to function correctly. The lymphatic system hosts the immune system and removes waste. When the lymphatic system lacks adequate water, it slows down. The slow movement of lymph contributes to a buildup of irritants and triggers the histamine response. More mucus is produced, resulting in more swelling and edema, and we suffer a cascade of uncomfortable effects.

The key to solving a chronic allergy problem is not allowing histamine to be produced in the first place. When you drink enough water, your body efficiently removes wastes via the lymphatic system (no histamine-triggering response occurs) and the immune system is able to work optimally. An additional positive effect is that the toxins stored in your muscles (that result in stiffness and fatigue) are likewise quickly carried away by a well-hydrated lymphatic system.

Now let's take a look at how water is related to obesity. When your body is dehydrated, it will do everything it can to hold on to water. Some of the excess weight in obesity is water being hoarded by your body. When you drink water regularly, your body gets the message that it is safe to release the excess water, it does release it, and pounds come off.

A second problem related to obesity is overeating, and this can occur when you mistake the sensation of thirst for the sensation of hunger, two sensations that can feel very similar. We also make a mistake when we think we are thirsty only when our mouths are dry. The key to avoiding overeating is to drink water before eating food. When you feel hungry, drink a glass or two of water. If you are still hungry 30 minutes later, go ahead and eat, because your sensation truly was hunger. You may well find, however, that you are no longer feeling that sensation—so you won't overeat because you're thirsty!

Water is of primary importance in so many of our bodies' functions that entire books are devoted to the topic. Consider a few more reasons that our bodies need adequate water:

§ Dehydration can interfere with sex-hormone production, resulting in impotence and low (or no) libido.

§ Dehydration makes PMS, menstrual cramps and hot flashes more severe.

§ Water makes the immune system more efficient and therefore better able to fight infections and cancer.

§ Water helps prevent memory loss associated with aging, reducing the risk of Alzheimer's disease, multiple sclerosis, Parkinson's disease and amyotrophic lateral sclerosis (ALS), or Lou Gehrig's disease.

§ Proper hydration helps reduce stress, anxiety and depression because water is directly involved in the effective manufacture of all neurotransmitters, including serotonin.

§ Water, the very best lubricating laxative, helps prevents constipation.

You can get more information about these and other essential functions of water by consulting Additional Wellness Resources in the back pages of this book.

## The Metaphysics of Water

Water is not only a life force for our planet and its inhabitants; it is also a symbol of purification—physically and spiritually. Its life-giving, spiritual nature runs throughout many of the world's religious cultures. It is used in ritual washings performed in several faiths, including Christianity, Judaism, Hinduism, Islam, Shinto and Taoism. Partial or total immersion in water is central to rituals such as baptism in Christianity and mikvah in Judaism. Several faiths prepare water for religious purposes, with blessings and prayer. This holy water is believed to have healing properties—as do certain bodies of water, according to some religions.

Japanese researcher Masaru Emoto has explored the connection between the resonance of water and the resonance of our thoughts. His hypothesis is that water, like all of creation, is energy, and that it can be affected by other energy sources. He set out to prove that water responds differently to positive or negative thoughts. Emoto collected water-droplet samples from around the world and exposed them to either positive or negative vibrations in the form of words, prayer and music. He then froze the droplets and photographed the crystals they produced. The water exposed to positive thoughts or energy created gorgeous crystals with unbelievable designs. The water exposed to negative thoughts created undefined, malformed and ugly crystals. With water such a huge component of life on this planet, and our world so full of negative thoughts and statements—"You're a fool; I hate you," "You'll never succeed"—what might that negativity be doing to our bodies? Something to ponder.

## Personal Stories

At age 26, Enkae Chang knew that something had to change. At 5 feet 8 and 255 pounds, he was clinically obese. He felt unmotivated and unhappy with his life. Enkae made a commitment to transform his unhealthy lifestyle. He enlisted the help of a personal and lifestyle coach, who taught him how to eat, move and live differently. Enkae started working out daily at the gym. *And he drank more than one gallon of water every day.*

Today, at age 28, Enkae is more than 90 pounds lighter, and he looks and feels great! He continues to drink a gallon of water a day. His energy is boundless, he feels more self-confident, and he is ready to build the real estate business of his dreams. He also hopes to become a motivational speaker and personal trainer so that he can help others. Enkae will tell you that his successful weight loss is directly related to his commitment to drink lots of water, which enabled his body to rid itself of years of stored toxins and fat.

Although not everyone needs a daily gallon of water, it's a formula that works well for Enkae and makes it possible for his body to work more efficiently. It keeps his unhealthy food cravings at bay and enhances his physical performance. Enkae has encouraging words for others: "Just make the simple change of drinking more water. You will be amazed at the positive response in your body!"

The signals we get to drink more water can be subtle or intense. Cori Colombe is a certified holistic health counselor who now works at YWC as a wellness advocate. Her own story of healing reveals the power of hydration. As a teenager, she lived in a very hot climate and trained hard as a gymnast. Her diet was much better than that of the average American teenager; however, she needed more and better nutrients to sustain the kind of athletic training required for a competitive gymnast. Cori also did not know about the

importance of hydration for wellness and athletic performance, so she was not diligent about getting the amount of
water required for her body's specific needs. It was during
this time that Cori began to have migraine headaches.

In her early 20s Cori started taking prescription medicine
to prevent her migraines. Yet the migraines grew worse, and
they began to occur more frequently—four or five times a
week. By her late 20s she was addicted to large doses of these
prescription medications. When she tried to stop taking the
meds, she would experience "rebound migraines" that were
intensely painful. The pain became so severe that she could
no longer effectively do her job, so she had to quit work. Cori
could no longer function in life. She felt miserable and
trapped.

She met a woman very close to her own age who was dealing with similar issues. This woman told Cori that she had
experienced a stroke because of the large doses of pain meds
she had been taking. This encounter affected Cori so deeply
that she immediately quit taking all of her own pain meds
"cold turkey"—a drastic decision that would leave her in
agony.

It was on Christmas Eve, several months after she had
stopped taking the meds, that Cori reached her breaking
point. She was beyond miserable—she felt like giving up. Her
body was stressed and exhausted, and Cori was in so much
pain that she wanted to die. She and her husband decided to
look for an acupuncturist, a healing modality that she had not
yet tried. They opened the phone book and found Your
Wellness Connection. Cori came in and, with treatment, got

some relief. This was the beginning of her journey toward wellness.

Cori sought guidance through prayer and the counsel of wellness professionals, and little by little she began to make changes in her lifestyle. One of the biggest and most significant changes for her was drinking adequate water and eating more hydrating foods, such as fruits and veggies. She would drink more water than usual if she was working out hard or if it was hot outside. She also began to limit her intake of unhealthy foods, especially those with a dehydrating effect. And she worked to decrease the stress in her daily life.

Today Cori has no migraine headaches. She says, "Hydration is definitely one of the keys. If I don't drink enough water, I always notice the side effects—maybe not immediately, but always within a day or two. Drinking water helps flush out all the toxins that accumulate in our bodies. And adequate hydration enhances the functioning of every single bodily system."

Cori encourages us to be gentle with ourselves as we learn. There is so much information out there, and it can be conflicting and confusing. When she tried a change that didn't work for her, she simply accepted that some things work for some people and not for others, and she moved on. She did a lot of research, and she kept what worked for her and released what didn't, with no judgment and no drama. Cori's approach was not "all or nothing"; rather, she believed that if she learned even one helpful thing from reading an entire book, then it was a good investment of her time. Having walked a healing path of her own, today Cori is an excellent support for others who are seeking wellness.

Ann Pai's health journey did not start out with water, but over time it has become the hub of her health. In the early 2000s, Ann, in her early 30s at the time, began seeing a counselor about a compulsive eating disorder. She'd had weight issues and hints of this disorder since her teenage years. She had tried the typical doctor's "one sheet" diet—you know, when your doctor hands you a sheet of paper and says, "Eat these things and not those, and you'll lose all your weight." If there was a fad diet, she had tried that too.

In 2001 Ann's older sister, who had battled severe morbid obesity, passed away after being hospitalized with complicated health issues—many of them related to her weight, which had reached 550 pounds. Ann began to process her sister's death and her own journey toward wellness by writing. She also continued to try different diet plans, including Weight Watchers. The best lesson she took from her time on that program was the regimen of drinking at least eight glasses of water a day. But Weight Watchers also lets you substitute a diet soda for a glass of water, and since Ann was a diet-soda junkie, she enjoyed that part of the plan.

When she began adding water and eventually replacing the soda with water, however, she began to notice tremendous differences. The first change was that her mood swings disappeared, as did her headaches and migraines. The water helped take the edge off the consistent, low-level anxiety and stress she felt. She also began sleeping better. The most significant change was that she could move! She had much more energy, and her body felt lubricated; she found that she could move more easily because of the water.

This set off a chain reaction in her life and wellness path. Ann changed the way she thought about health and what she needed to make her body move and be more efficient. She began to listen to the feedback her body was giving her and was determined to meet those needs more healthfully. She says, "When you begin to see your 'medicine cabinet' as water, healthy food, moving your body and getting adequate sleep, you don't seek out nutrient-poor foods and other toxic habits to meet your so-called needs."

For Ann, the connection between hydration and total mind-body-spirit well-being was now clear. She realized that since she was a teenager, a big part of her struggle had been that she was dehydrated. She felt a little sad about all those wasted years, all the negative self-talk and beating up on herself. But she was also grateful that she'd finally had this "aha" moment and changed her life.

With the increased activity made possible by the greater energy she felt from being fully hydrated, Ann has reached a comfortable weight without restrictive dieting. She published a book about her sister and her own journey in 2006. She has become a triathlete and avid trail runner. Ann always drinks plenty of water each day, and no soda. She makes it fun by using bendy straws! She drinks extra water in the winter, when she feels dry because of heated indoor air; in the summer, when she spends more time outside; and whenever she puts in a hard workout. If she ever feels she hasn't drunk enough water, instead of admonishing herself with, "Go get some water!" she gently says to herself, "Honey, protect yourself." Her entire approach to health and well-being is about supporting her body and giving it what it needs—starting with water.

⌒

~

## Practical Tips for Your Journey

YWC wellness advocate Shelly Murray recommends being mindful (but not obsessive!) about these tips:

1. Consider making it a goal to drink enough water every day to maintain proper hydration. (Divide your body weight in pounds by two; that figure indicates the number of ounces of water to drink daily. For example, if you weigh 150 pounds, dividing by two is 75. Drink 75 ounces of water each day.) If you are very sedentary, or if you eat lots of hydrating fruits and veggies every day, you may need less. If you are very active, or if you work outside in hot weather, you may need more. If you are flying or going to a warmer climate, or if you keep the temperature very warm in your house, your requirements may also be higher.

2. When you go to bed at night, fill a 16-ounce glass with water. Set it by your bed. When you awake in the morning, drink this water immediately. This will help flush your kidneys and replace any water you lost during the night.

3. Next, fill a large glass with half the remaining water you need to consume for the day, and drink the entire glass of water during midmorning.

4. Refill your glass with the remaining water you need to drink that day, and finish it during midafternoon. Thus, you have your minimum daily requirement of water consumed before dinner, and you avoid the problem of wak-

~

ing in the night to urinate, which often occurs when you drink lots of water in the evening.

5. Try not to drink 30 minutes to one hour before or after meals so that you do not dilute the acid your stomach needs for proper digestion and absorption of nutrients. If you must have a drink with your meal, make it room-temperature water (no ice) and keep it to four ounces or less. Drinking a full glass of water just before meals does not help with weight loss, but it does hamper digestion of key nutrients that your body needs to function well.

6. Do not count flavored water, juices, soft drinks, coffee, tea or any other beverages toward your daily ounces of water. And remember that drinks such as coffee, caffeinated tea and alcohol will dehydrate you. A good practice is to drink a full glass of water after each dehydrating drink.

7. Drink the purest water you can get. Tap water may be safer (and it's certainly cheaper!) than bottled water because it is regulated according to certain quality standards. You can request a water-quality report from your local water utility. If you choose to filter water, there are several inexpensive options, including Brita and PUR. If your budget allows for it, you may want to install a filtration system either for a single source of filtered water or at the point of entry to your house, filtering all water that comes into your home. At Your Wellness Connection, we use a filtration system from Boresow's Water Company.

8. Consider carrying your water in a reusable metal (which I prefer to aluminum) bottle such as the SIGG bottle. They are washable, durable and recyclable, and they have an

internal coating that is resistant to stains, smells and bacterial buildup. These bottles are thoroughly tested to ensure absolutely no leaching (unlike many plastic water bottles), so they are 100 percent safe. They are also eco-friendly and creatively designed, which makes them fun to carry!

9. When you are experiencing a craving or intense hunger, consider that you may be dehydrated. Drink a big glass of water and wait 30 minutes to one hour to see if you are still hungry. This is an important strategy for children too. When they come home from school ravenous, give them a big glass of water. If they're still hungry after half an hour, go ahead and serve them a healthy snack.

10. Remember that your body will take some time to get used to being fully hydrated, so don't expect instant changes. It takes cells time to regenerate, and as we grow healthy new cells in an environment of adequate hydration, we feel better and better.

11. Experiment, see how you feel, and keep a journal of what you observe about yourself as you make this lifestyle change. You will likely notice your mood lifting, your energy increasing and your athletic ability improving, along with many other health benefits, as your body utilizes the water you are drinking for myriad life functions.

12. As always, if you have any health concerns or feel, for any reason, that drinking more water could be harmful to you, see a physician (a D.C., M.D. or D.O.) to run some tests. Discuss your concerns, your current lifestyle practices and any medications or nutritional supplements you may be taking, and then decide together what is the best

course of action for you to follow.

13. Remember that this is a life journey. Take a long-term view. Some days you won't get all the water you need; other days you will. Be gentle and patient with yourself, and do your best. Little by little, step by step, good choice by good choice, you will transform your life!

## Your Space

Use this page to make notes and write your own reflections on drinking to your health.

_____

_____

_____

_____

_____

_____

_____

_____

_____

_____

_____

_____

_____

_____

Epilogue

# Tie Your Wellness Together

# Epilogue

～

"When health is absent, wisdom cannot reveal itself,
art cannot become manifest, strength cannot fight,
wealth becomes useless,
and intelligence cannot be applied."

—Herophilus

This book began with the assertion that wellness is attainable on a shoestring budget. Five of the practices—rest, reflect and rejuvenate; breathe deeply; move your body; free your space; and drink to your health—include many suggestions that are absolutely free. The other two—go for the greens, and the combination eat from the sea and enjoy the sun—have simple requirements like adapting your grocery list, using the cash you already budget for food to make nutritious choices when you shop, or just spending a little more time outdoors. We really can live healthier lives without spending a lot of money! The key is intentionally choosing wellness every day and practicing these lifestyle choices.

It's important to realize that it's not one single change that makes you well. It's tying all of them together—kind of like when you host a party. You want the decor to feel welcoming. You want to have plenty of space and chairs. You want the right music, the right food, the right blend of activities and people. If one of these things is off, the whole party can turn out very differently than you planned, or it can become work and no fun at all. Similarly, you want the healthy lifestyle practices outlined in this book working together in order to benefit your overall wellness.

～

How do you tie them all together? Trust your spirit to guide you as you make choices to maintain your body's health. Ask yourself where the most important place is for you to begin making a healthy change, and then trust your own guidance to make one change at a time, at a pace that feels comfortable to you. Your wellness journey may not look like anyone else's journey, and that is just fine.

Remember that, on average, it takes 18 to 36 months to move from disease to wellness, so be patient! Your health likely did not get to where it is today overnight, and you need to allow yourself grace, gentleness and time as you grow stronger and move into wellness. Step by step, you will absolutely transform your life. *I pray that your wellness choices connect to the life of your dreams.*

# Additional Wellness Resources

These resources can help guide you as you continue your wellness journey.

### Chapter 1: Rest, Reflect and Rejuvenate

Michael Bernard Beckwith, Agape International Spiritual Center: *www.agapelive.com* (a source of ideas about the power of reflection and ways to rejuvenate your spirit)

Centerpointe Meditation: *www.centerpointe.com* (tools to help rest your mind)

Chicken Soup for the Soul: *www.chickensoup.com* (stories that can rejuvenate your heart and spirit)

Sonia Choquette. *The Answer Is Simple … Love Yourself, Live Your Spirit!* Hay House, 2008. *www.soniachoquette.com*

*Daily Word*®: *www.dailyword.com* (a daily reading to allow for reflection with your spirit)

Hay House: *www.hayhouse.com* (tools to help you focus on positive thoughts and actions)

I Am a Miracle Foundation: *www.iamamiracle.com* (its stories can rejuvenate your heart and spirit)

Rev. Joel Osteen: *www.joelosteen.com* (for inspirational, spirit-filled living)

Rhythmic Medicine: *www.rhythmicmedicine.com* (tools to calm your mind, body and spirit)

Unity: *www.unity.org* (resources and tools to reconnect and rejuvenate your spirit; also a resource for retreats)


## Chapter 2: Breathe Deeply

Art of Living: *www.artofliving.org* (for lessons on *how* to breathe)

Ciardha Carey: *www.breathmechanics.com*

Mary Omwake: *www.maryomwake.com* (resources and tools from a visionary leader on meditating and connecting to spirit and breath)

Mark Stanton Welch: *www.markstantonwelch.com*

Jill Tupper: *www.jilltupper.com*


## Chapter 3: Move Your Body

James L. Chestnut, D.C. *The 14 Foundational Premises for the Scientific and Philosophical Validation of the Chiropractic Wellness Paradigm.* Global Self Health Corp., 2003. *www.thewellnesspractice.com*

Sean Foy, *The 10-Minute Total Body Breakthrough.* New York, NY: Workman Publishing Company, Inc., 2009.

International Yang Family Tai Chi Chuan Association: *www.yangfamilytaichi.com/home*

Iyengar yoga: *www.iynaus.org*

Christiane Northrup, M.D.: *The Wisdom of Menopause: Creating Physical and Mental Health and Healing During the Change.* New York, NY: Bantam Dell, 2001.

*Women's Bodies, Women's Wisdom: Creating Physical and Emotional Health and Healing.* New York, NY: Bantam Dell, 2006.

*www.drnorthrup.com* (resources on physical and emotional health issues specific to women throughout their lives)

B.J. Palmer, D.C.: *www.upcspine.com/greenbooks1.htm* or *www.facebook.com/group.php?gid=14836649660* (learn about the father of chiropractic and his work at these sites)

## Chapter 4: Free Your Space

Terah Kathryn Collins: *The Western Guide to Feng Shui: Room by Room.* Carlsbad, CA: Hay House, 1999.

Feng Shui: *www.fengshui.about.com*

The Hoffman Institute International: *www.hoffman institute.com*; "Negative Love," *A Path to Personal Freedom and Love,* www.hoffmaninstitute.org/process/path-to-personal-freedom/4.html

Karen Kingston. *Clear Your Clutter With Feng Shui.* New York, NY: Broadway Books, 1999.

Denise Linn. *Sacred Space: Enhancing the Energy of Your Home and Office.* London: Rider & Co., 2005.

Mehmet Oz, M.D.: *www.realage.com/gicenter/intro.aspx*

Sunlighten Infrared Saunas: *www.sunlightsaunas.com* (for decluttering your body by removing toxins)

## Chapter 5: Go for the Greens

Johnna Albi and Catherine Walthers. *Greens Glorious Greens: More Than 140 Ways to Prepare All Those Great-Tasting, Super-Healthy, Beautiful Leafy Greens.* New York, NY: St. Martin's Griffin, 1996.

Victoria Boutenko. *Green for Life.* Canada: Raw Family Publishing, 2005.

Centers for Disease Control and Prevention: "Eat a Variety of Fruits and Vegetables Every Day," */www.fruitsandveggies-matter.gov/*

James L. Chestnut, D.C.: *The Innate Diet and Natural Hygiene.* Global Self Health Corp., 2004. *www.thewellnesspractice.com*

Brian Clement, Ph.D., Hippocrates Health Institute: *www.hippocratesinst.org* (tools, resources and on-site experiences for healthy eating and wellness practices)

The Daily Green, "Top 12 Foods to Eat Organic": *www.thedailygreen.com/healthy-eating/eat-safe/Dirty-Dozen-Foods*

Environmental Working Group, "Shopper's Guide to Pesticides": *www.foodnews.org/fulllist.php*

David Heber, M.D., Ph.D. *What Color Is Your Diet?* New York, NY: Harper Paperbacks, 2002.

Vita-Mix: *www.vitamix.com* (kitchen tools and recipes for greening up your life)

~

Your Wellness Connection: *www.yourwellnessconnection.com*

## Chapter 6: Eat From the Sea—and Enjoy the Sun!

Innate Choice: The Science of Wellness Nutrition: *www.innat-echoice.com* (to find research on omega-3; also a supplier)

Mercola.com: Take Control of Your Health: *www.mercola.com* (resources and research on many health topics; written by a medical doctor)

## Chapter 7: Drink to Your Health

John Douillard, Ph.D. *Body, Mind, and Sport: The Mind-Body Guide to Lifelong Health, Fitness and Your Personal Best.* New York, NY: Three Rivers Press, 2001.

Boresow's Water Company: *www.boresow-water.com*

Masaru Emoto: *www.masaru-emoto.net/english/e_ome_home.html*

Steve Meyerowitz. *Water—the Ultimate Cure: Discover Why Water Is the Most Important Ingredient in Your Diet and Find Out Which Water Is Right for You.* Great Barrington, MA: Sproutman Publications, 2000.

# Endnotes

## Chapter 1: Rest, Reflect and Rejuvenate

[1] Wayne W. Dyer, Ph.D. *The Power of Intention.* Carlsbad, CA: Hay House, 2005. *www.drwaynedyer.com*

## Chapter 2: Breathe Deeply

[1] Thich Nhat Hanh. *Meditations on the Present Moment.* CD. One Spirit, 2000. *www.plumvillage.org*

## Chapter 3: Move Your Body

[1] Mayo Clinic. "Aerobic Exercise: Top 10 Reasons to Get Physical." February 14, 2009. <https://www.mayoclinic.com/health/aerobic-exercise/EP00002> (Accessed January 2010).

[2] Mayo Clinic. "Strength Training: Get Stronger, Leaner and Healthier." July 4, 2008. <https://www.mayoclinic.com/health/strength-training/HQ01710> (Accessed January 2010).

[3] American Heart Association. "Target Heart Rates." <http://www.americanheart.org/presenter.jhtml?identifier=4736> (Accessed January 2010).

[4] Cleveland Clinic. "Pulse and Target Heart Rate." <http://my.clevelandclinic.org/heart/prevention/exercise/pulsethr.aspx> (Accessed January 2010).

## Chapter 5: Go for the Greens

[1] Institute for Integrative Nutrition: *www.integrative nutrition.com*

[2] Tanya Edwards, M.D., Med. "Inflammation, Pain, and Chronic Disease: An Integrative Approach to Treatment and Prevention." *Alternative Therapies in Health and Medicine.* Vol. 11, No. 6, November 2005.

## Chapter 6: Eat From the Sea—and Enjoy the Sun!

[1] Bernandine Healy, M.D. "From Fish Oil to Medicine." *US News & World Report* August 2008.

[2] Andrew Weil, M.D. "Q & A Library: Balancing Omega-3 and Omega-6." Februray 22, 2007. Drweil.com, 2010. <http://www.drweil.com/drw/u/QAA400149/balancing-omega-3-and-omega-6.html>

[3] National Institutes of Health. "Medical Encyclopedia: Vitamin D." March 7, 2009. <http://www.nlm.nih.gov/medlineplus/ency/article/002405.htm> (Accessed January 2010). "Dietary Supplement Fact Sheet: Vitamin D." November 13, 2009. <http://dietary-supplements.info.nih.gov/factsheets/vitamind.asp> (Accessed January 2010).

## Chapter 7: Drink to Your Health

[1] John Douillard, Ph.D. *Perfect Health for Kids: Ten Ayurvedic Health Secrets Every Parent Must Know.* Berkeley, CA: North Atlantic Books, 2004.

[2] F. Batmanghelidj, M.D. *Water for Health, for Healing, for Life: You're Not Sick, You're Thirsty!* New York, NY: Grand Central Publishing, 2003.

# Acknowledgements

**From Michelle Robin:**

Thank you, God, for giving me a passion for wellness and guiding me on this journey.

For all of you who contribute to my life and fuel my passion in so many different, but all impactful, ways:

To all my clients who have allowed me to share in your wellness journeys: You mean the world to me. Thank you for sharing your lives with me. Extra-special thanks go to Gina Danner, Lee Harris, Laura Lenehan, Eddie Penrice, Linda Pfingsten, Patti Phillips, Angela Rizzo, Karen Zecy, Fred Pryor, Francene Lisle, Ann Pai and Marlene Sohl, who graciously shared their experiences for the purpose of getting this book into the world.

To my editor, Shelly Kramer, thank you for providing me with attention to detail and professional support that took this book to a higher level.

To Rebecca Korphage, thank you for giving of your talents and helping me round out this book and provide a fuller experience for the reader.

To Rev. Roxanne Renée Grant, thank you for helping me capture the essence of this book.

To all my team members at Your Wellness Connection, current and past, who have walked this journey with me: You will never know how grateful I am! You guys are amazing—every single day!

To all my coaches and mentors: Thank you, Ron and Linda Pfingsten, Dr. John and Carol Lakin, Dr. Richard Yennie, Pat

Khan, Cindy Currie, Rev. Mary Omwake, Dr. Jack Sibley, Sally Smith, Bill and Vicki Reisler, Rev. Patricia Bass, Dr. Tom Hill and Dr. Janice Hughes for the wealth of guidance and wisdom you have shared and continue to share with me.

To my colleagues at the Helzberg Entrepreneurial Mentoring Program, and especially to our fearless leader, Barnett Helzberg Jr., thank you for inspiring me.

To the greatest group of businesswomen in the universe— the *Kansas City Business Journal*'s "Women Who Mean Business"—thank you for pushing me to be the best I can be.

To my Translucent U Team—Cuky Harvey, Sonia Choquette, Karl and Kyle Peschke, Debra Graves, Mark Welch, Kimo, Brad Easton, Sabrina Tully and Crystal Jenkins—thank you for allowing me to grow in your sandbox.

To Unity, which is not only my publisher but is also a great friend to me and to all the communities it serves: Your organization and the message you spread are very dear to my heart. And thanks especially to Dr. Charlotte Shelton for her support.

Finally, to my biggest fan, C.J., thank you for your patience, love and acceptance.

**From Roxanne Renée Grant:**

My heartfelt thanks to:

God, the Source of all that is Life in me and of the Grace that sustains me each day.

Dr. Michelle Robin, for the opportunity to share in birthing this book.

# Acknowledgements

〜

Those I interviewed, for entrusting your stories to me; it was an honor.

My beloved sons, Truman and Jay, for sacrificing "mommy time" so that I could write.

Doty, for believing in me on days when I doubt, and for walking with me no matter where the path leads.

Amy, for providing practical help, great meals and sanctuary.

Josh, for offering me a humorous perspective and for insisting that I take your chair.

Drs. Corey Priest, Steven Timmer and Amanda Toney, for ongoing nutritional guidance and excellent chiropractic care.

Eric, for brilliant business coaching and for running beside me every step of that last mile. It was your friendship that got me across this finish line on time.

〜

# About the Authors

**DR. MICHELLE ROBIN** has been involved in wellness in the Kansas City, Missouri, metropolitan area for 28 years. She is the chief wellness officer (CWO) and founder of Your Wellness Connection, P.A. She graduated from Cleveland Chiropractic College in 1991 and opened her own practice in 1992. In 2001 her vision to change people's lives by connecting them to holistic wellness practices and treatments led her to build a state-of-the-art healing facility. She leads a team of 30 members and operates one of the most successful healing centers in the nation, focusing on integrative healing disciplines such as chiropractic, Chinese medicine, massage therapy, functional medicine, counseling, nutritional counseling and coaching, wellness coaching and movement arts.

Dr. Robin and her dedication and service to the Kansas City community have been recognized in many ways, including national recognition by the Master's Circle as Chiropractor of the Year (2007) and by the House of Menuha with its Community Service Award (2005); designation as one of the *Kansas City Business Journal*'s Women Who Mean Business (2003); and designation by the *Kansas City Small Business Monthly* as one of the "Top 25 Under 25 Small Businesses" (2002). She is a regular contributing writer to *Flourish! Magazine*, a publication for businesswomen, and a regular contributor to other community publications focusing on health and wellness.

Giving back to the community and to the world is very important to Dr. Robin. She has held board positions for a variety of not-for-profit organizations, including KC Free Health Clinic; House of Menuha, an organization dedicated to providing women a quiet space for rest and renewal; and SAFEHOME, an organization dedicated to ending domestic violence and providing a home for women and children in crisis. She currently serves on the board of the Menorah Legacy Foundation, the Advisory Board for KC Free Health Clinic, and the board of Turning Point.

Since 2003 Dr. Robin has been a member of the Helzberg Entrepreneurial Mentoring Program (HEMP), an organization started by Barnett Helzberg Jr. HEMP supports local entrepreneurs through peer-to-peer mentoring. Dr. Robin actively seeks ways to share her wellness message through local and national speaking engagements as well as collaborative efforts with other wellness practitioners. She also assists many corporations with the development of wellness programs to keep employees well and thriving. Dr. Robin's other interests include spirituality, travel, reading, biking and basketball. She recently competed in her third triathlon and is committed to striving to be in the best shape of her life.

Dr. Robin has a vision to enhance wellness in people's lives by empowering them to connect to themselves and get back to basic wellness practices. She is a passionate and committed international wellness advocate, and her personal mission statement reads, "I connect and inspire people to live well." You may contact her at *www.yourwellnessconnection.com*.


**REV. ROXANNE RENÉE GRANT**, who has a master's of divinity, with an emphasis in pastoral care and counseling, was ordained in 1994. She has worked in ministry for the past 19 years, serving in a variety of ministry settings among diverse groups. She has experience as a pastor, chaplain, public speaker, spiritual counselor, mental wellness coach, wellness lifestyle trainer, writer, vocal artist and voice-over artist.

In addition to her professional experience, Rev. Grant has personal experience of healing through a combination of traditional and alternative approaches, and she maintains her own wellness through lifestyle commitments. She speaks to large and small groups in her trademark seminar entitled "Living Beyond Depression: Seven Daily Lifestyle Choices to Support Wellness and Reduce Risk of Relapse." You may contact Rev. Grant at *www.roxannerenee.com.*